The Blood Sugar Solution to Mental Health

Unlocking the Link Between Blood Sugar and Mental Health Recovery

---

Greg Doney

Paperback ISBN: 978-1-7646377-3-2

Hardcover ISBN: 978-1-7646377-5-6

Epub ISBN: 978-1-7646377-4-9

Medical Disclaimer

This book and its contents are provided for informational purposes only. The author and publisher make no representations or warranties regarding the accuracy, completeness, or applicability of the content. They disclaim all liability for any errors, omissions, or inconsistencies that may be present.

The content in this book is not intended to diagnose, treat, cure, or prevent any condition or disease. It is not a substitute for professional medical advice, diagnosis, or treatment. Always consult a licensed healthcare professional before making any changes to your health regimen or treatment plan. The use of this book implies your understanding and acceptance of this disclaimer.

First edition

Contents

Introduction

Overview of Blood Sugar and Mental Health

In recent years, scientific research has increasingly illuminated the powerful role that blood sugar regulation plays in mental health. Though we typically think of blood sugar as primarily relevant to diabetes or metabolic disorders, it also has a real impact on mood, cognitive function, and emotional resilience. *The Blood Sugar Solution to Mental Health* brings together the latest science and practical strategies to help readers understand how blood sugar stability contributes to better mental health.

Central to this book is a simple but often overlooked idea: managing blood sugar is not just about physical health; it is also a crucial element in supporting a stable, resilient mind. Blood sugar fluctuations affect our emotional states and energy levels on a daily basis. When blood sugar spikes and then crashes, a typical result of consuming high-sugar or refined foods, these swings can lead to mood shifts, irritability, brain fog, and fatigue. Over time, they can contribute to more severe mental health issues, including depression and anxiety.

This book provides readers with a comprehensive guide to achieving balanced blood sugar and understanding its effects on mental well-being. By adopting simple yet impactful lifestyle changes, you will discover how to improve your mood, clarity, and energy naturally and sustainably.

Why Blood Sugar Matters

Blood sugar imbalances can create a range of mental health symptoms that are easy to miss or dismiss. You may notice irritability, lack of focus, cravings, or fatigue, but not immediately connect these to blood sugar fluctuations. Yet these issues are often directly related to the highs and lows of glucose levels, which in turn affect the brain's access to stable energy.

When blood sugar levels are high, there is a temporary increase in energy and alertness. However, as the body works to lower these levels, a sharp decline in blood sugar often follows. This drop, or "crash," can leave you feeling lethargic, anxious, or moody. Understanding and addressing these fluctuations is essential, not just for physical health, but for emotional balance and mental clarity as well.

This book will help you recognise the role blood sugar plays in your mental health journey. Through clear explanations, practical tips, and research-backed advice, you will learn to recognise signs of blood sugar imbalances and discover how stabilising these levels can enhance your mental and emotional well-being.

Introducing Key Contributors

Leading voices in the fields of nutrition, psychiatry, and metabolic health support the guidance offered in this book. The research and findings from these experts form the scientific backbone of the strategies and insights provided here:

- **Dr Julia Rucklidge** is a clinical psychologist whose groundbreaking research on nutrition and mental health highlights how blood sugar regulation and nutrient intake influence mood disorders.
- **Dr Felice Jacka** is known as a pioneer in nutritional psychiatry. Her studies underscore the importance of diet in mental health, particularly the role that blood sugar stability plays in managing depression and anxiety.
- **Dr David Ludwig** is an endocrinologist and researcher specialising in obesity and metabolic health. Dr Ludwig has shown that stabilising blood sugar through dietary choices can significantly support mental clarity and resilience.

- **Dr Shebani Sethi** is a psychiatrist and metabolic health expert whose research at Stanford's Metabolic Psychiatry Clinic focuses on the relationship between metabolic health and mental health, particularly how insulin resistance and inflammation impact mood and cognition.

These experts' work has significantly advanced our understanding of the connections between blood sugar and mental health, and their findings provide the scientific foundation for the strategies you will find throughout this book.

How to Use This Book

The Blood Sugar Solution to Mental Health is organised to be both educational and actionable. Each chapter offers background knowledge paired with practical steps, empowering you to take control of your blood sugar for improved mental well-being.

Foundational Knowledge: The opening chapters cover essential concepts, from understanding blood sugar's impact on mood to the role of key hormones like insulin and cortisol. These chapters set the stage for deeper exploration and help you understand the science behind the strategies.

Practical, Targeted Strategies: In subsequent chapters, you will find guidance on diet, sleep, exercise, and environmental factors that influence blood sugar and mental health. These chapters provide specific steps you can apply immediately, whether you are making minor adjustments to your diet, creating a sleep-supportive environment, or integrating stress management practices.

Personalised Approaches and Long-Term Success: Toward the end of the book, you will find resources to help you tailor blood sugar management to your lifestyle, track your progress, and build sustainable habits. These chapters also discuss how to adapt strategies for different life stages and situations, making it easier to maintain balanced blood sugar and mental well-being over the long term.

Every chapter is crafted to support you on your path to achieving mental clarity, emotional stability, and sustained energy through balanced blood sugar.

This book is not just a guide, it is a practical tool for anyone seeking a deeper understanding of how the foods they eat, the routines they follow, and the lifestyle they maintain impact their mind and body. By the end, you will have the knowledge and strategies to make meaningful changes, helping you feel better, think more clearly, and live a life of greater balance and resilience.

References

Rucklidge, J. J., & Kaplan, B. J. (2014). Broad-spectrum micronutrient treatment for attention-deficit/hyperactivity disorder: Rationale and evidence to date. *CNS Drugs*, 28(9), 775–785. https://doi.org/10.1007/s40263-014-0190-4

Jacka, F. N., O'Neil, A., Opie, R., Itsiopoulos, C., Cotton, S., Mohebbi, M., … & Berk, M. (2017). A randomised controlled trial of dietary improvement for adults with major depression (the "SMILES" trial). *BMC Medicine*, 15(1), 23.

Ludwig, D. S. (2016). *Always hungry? Conquer cravings, retrain your fat cells, and lose weight permanently*. Grand Central Life & Style.

Sethi, S. (2023). Metabolic psychiatry: Bridging metabolic and mental health. *Psychiatric Clinics of North America*, 46(3), 487–499.

Knüppel, A., Shipley, M. J., Llewellyn, C. H., & Brunner, E. J. (2017). Sugar intake from sweet food and beverages, common mental disorder and depression: Prospective findings from the Whitehall II study. *Scientific Reports*, 7, 6287.

Mantantzis, K., Schlaghecken, F., Sünram-Lea, S. I., & Maylor, E. A. (2019). Sugar rush or sugar crash? A meta-analysis of carbohydrate effects on mood. *Neuroscience & Biobehavioral Reviews*, 101, 45–67.

Chapter 1: The Sugar-Mood Connection

Understanding the Metabolic-Emotional Link

For many people struggling with anxiety, irritability, or persistent low mood, the culprit is not a psychiatric disorder requiring medication. It is a metabolic imbalance that shifts with each meal. The direct relationship between the sugar we eat, the stability of our blood sugar, and our emotional wellbeing is one of the most important connections in mental health, and one that mainstream psychiatry has been slow to take seriously.

When you consume foods high in sugar, they are rapidly broken down into glucose and flood the bloodstream. Your pancreas responds by releasing insulin — think of insulin as the key that unlocks cell doors, allowing glucose to enter and fuel your body. But when this process happens too quickly and too often, your body enters a cycle of spikes and crashes. These swings in blood sugar create noticeable shifts in mood, triggering feelings of anxiety, irritability, or exhaustion that can feel overwhelming and disconnected from diet.

This knowledge transforms diet from a cosmetic health concern into a core strategy for emotional stability and cognitive clarity.

How Blood Sugar Affects Your Brain

Your brain is extraordinarily dependent on a steady supply of glucose. Despite accounting for only 2 per cent of your body weight, your brain consumes approximately 20 per cent of your total glucose supply. Unlike your muscles or liver, which can store glucose as glycogen for later use, your brain has virtually no reserves. This makes it acutely vulnerable to blood sugar fluctuations.

When your blood sugar remains stable, your brain receives consistent fuel and functions optimally; you feel calm, focused, and emotionally regulated. When blood sugar drops sharply, your brain becomes metabolically starved. Your body interprets this as a threat and releases stress hormones like adrenaline and cortisol. These hormones trigger the classic symptoms of a "sugar crash": anxiety, irritability, fatigue, and an intense craving for quick carbohydrates.

Over time, frequent blood sugar swings rewire your emotional baseline. The constant cycling of feast and famine teaches your nervous system to be hypervigilant, always anticipating the next crisis. This pattern, repeated day after day, contributes directly to mood disorders, anxiety, and depression in vulnerable individuals.

What Research Has Revealed

Research has shown clear links between high sugar consumption and mental health problems. Dr Anika Knüppel's landmark Whitehall II Study tracked thousands of participants over time and found that individuals with high sugar intake were significantly more likely to develop mood disorders, including depression. The findings were striking: while sugar offered a brief energy boost, it ultimately worsened mood instability and deepened depressive symptoms over time.

Dr Konstantinos Mantantzis and colleagues conducted separate research examining what researchers call the "sugar crash" effect. Their work confirmed what many people experience intuitively: while sugar might briefly elevate mood and energy, it is quickly followed by a sharp decline in both. This crash leads to worsened irritability and fatigue, a cycle that is particularly harmful to those already vulnerable to emotional dysregulation.

The Interoception Factor: Why You Are Unique

A key 2025 study revealed something remarkable about how blood sugar affects mood. The research used continuous glucose monitoring, tiny sensors that track blood sugar throughout the day, combined with moment-to-moment mood tracking. The findings challenged conventional thinking: lower blood glucose was indeed linked to worsened mood, but the relationship was entirely mediated by something unexpected, your *conscious awareness of hunger*.

This ability to accurately sense what is happening inside your body is called **interoception**. Your nervous system constantly monitors internal signals: heart rate, hunger, temperature, metabolic state. Some people perceive these signals clearly and accurately. Others misread them. The study showed that individuals with high interoceptive accuracy, those who reliably recognised when their blood sugar was dropping, experienced significantly fewer mood fluctuations, even during identical glucose swings.

Individuals with poor interoceptive awareness, by contrast, consistently misinterpreted a glucose dip as a psychological threat. Their brains amplified the emotional response disproportionately, turning a normal metabolic event into what felt like a crisis. In conditions like depression and anxiety, this interoceptive system may be essentially impaired. Normal physiological fluctuations get misread as existential dangers, triggering cascading emotional responses.

This finding offers hope. By stabilising your blood sugar through dietary strategies, you accomplish two things simultaneously: you reduce how often these metabolic fluctuations occur, and over time, your brain's interoceptive alarm system gradually recalibrates. You become better at interpreting your body's signals accurately.

Recognising Your Symptoms

Blood sugar imbalances manifest subtly but persistently. Learning to identify them in your daily life is the first step toward understanding the blood sugar-mood connection:

- **Irritability and mood swings** often appear after eating high-sugar foods. You may feel calm one moment, then suddenly irritable or anxious without obvious external cause.
- **Anxiety and nervousness** frequently accompany blood sugar crashes. When glucose drops, your body releases stress hormones to stabilise levels, creating feelings of restlessness and unease.

- **Brain fog and fatigue** represent your brain's metabolic struggle. The temporary "high" after eating sugary foods gives way to profound fatigue and cognitive haziness as glucose plummets.
- **Intense cravings** for sweets or carbohydrates emerge from the body's desperate attempt to restore blood sugar quickly, creating a cycle difficult to break.

Dr Sara Gottfried, an expert in hormonal balance, emphasises that these symptoms are deeply tied to hormonal shifts triggered by blood sugar dysregulation. When blood glucose rises sharply, your pancreas releases large quantities of insulin to bring it down. This creates the rollercoaster effect that impacts both mood and energy. Awareness of these patterns helps you recognise the intimate connection between what you eat and how you feel emotionally.

Sugar and Your Brain's Reward System

Sugar is far more than a source of calories. It is a psychoactive substance that triggers the brain's reward pathways with neurobiological similarities to substance use. This process, called **dopamine dysregulation**, represents a crucial driver of both metabolic disease and mood disorders.

Ultra-processed foods containing refined sugars generate an opioid-like pleasure response via the **mesocorticolimbic reward system**, the same neural circuit activated by heroin. Repeated exposure triggers neuroadaptation within weeks. Chronically, this consumption produces **anhedonia**: the brain becomes incapable of experiencing pleasure from previously rewarding sources and requires progressively larger quantities of high-sugar foods to achieve the same effect.

This progression mirrors addiction precisely. When you consume high-sugar foods repeatedly, **dopamine D2 receptors** in your brain's reward centres become downregulated, reduced in number and sensitivity. This is identical to what occurs with cocaine, alcohol, and opioids. Your brain adapts by reducing its capacity to respond to the rewarding stimulus, requiring progressively larger doses to feel the same pleasure. You develop tolerance.

With downregulated dopamine receptors, you experience reduced pleasure from previously rewarding activities. Your motivational salience system becomes hyperfocused on food-related cues. Images of sweets, the smell of a bakery, or even thoughts of sugar trigger intense cravings and heightened reward anticipation. When you attempt to restrict sugar intake, to recover, withdrawal symptoms emerge: anxiety, irritability, dysphoria, and restlessness. This is not weakness. It is genuine neurochemistry requiring compassion, support, and often structured dietary approaches to overcome.

Another mechanism, called **cross-sensitisation**, links sugar consumption to anxiety and mood disorders. The repeated dopamine spikes from sugar gradually sensitise your entire reward system. Neutral stressors, frustrations, social challenges, minor disappointments, begin to produce disproportionate emotional reactivity and anxiety. Your brain, primed by chronic sugar use, interprets ordinary situations as threatening.

Understanding this neurobiological reality is essential: the difficulty you experience withdrawing from sugar is not merely a matter of willpower. It reflects genuine neurochemical adjustment. Recovery requires weeks to months as dopamine receptors normalise, a period during which you may feel anhedonic, low, and crave sugar intensely.

Key Takeaways

- Sugar consumption creates rapid spikes and crashes in blood glucose, triggering mood instability, anxiety, and fatigue.
- Your brain's ability to accurately perceive and interpret its own metabolic signals (called interoception) directly determines how dramatically blood sugar changes affect your emotions.
- High sugar consumption alters dopamine signalling in the brain's reward centres, producing addiction-like patterns of tolerance, withdrawal, and cross-sensitisation to other stressors.
- Stabilising blood sugar through dietary change addresses this cycle on two levels: reducing metabolic fluctuations and gradually recalibrating your brain's emotional alarm system.

- The research linking sugar to mood disorders is compelling and consistent; for many individuals with depression or anxiety, dietary change offers a clinically significant intervention.

Next Steps

Sugar is not a monolithic substance. Different types of sugar (glucose, fructose, sucrose, lactose) have vastly different effects on blood glucose and mental health. In Chapter 2, we examine the chemistry of sugar and carbohydrates, exploring which types of sugar most destabilise your mood and which dietary approaches can restore metabolic balance.

References

Knüppel, A., Shipley, M. J., Llewellyn, C. H., & Brunner, E. J. (2017). Sugar intake from sweet food and beverages, common mental disorder and depression: Prospective findings from the Whitehall II study. *Scientific Reports*, 7, 6287. https://doi.org/10.1038/srep42996

Mantantzis, K., Schlaghecken, F., Sünram-Lea, S. I., & Maylor, E. A. (2019). Sugar rush or sugar crash? A meta-analysis of carbohydrate effects on mood. *Neuroscience & Biobehavioral Reviews*, 101, 45–67. https://doi.org/10.1016/j.neubiorev.2019.03.016

Gottfried, S. (2013). *The hormone cure: Reclaim balance, sleep, sex drive, and vitality naturally with the Gottfried Protocol*. Scribner.

Avena, N. M., Rada, P., & Hoebel, B. G. (2008). Evidence for sugar addiction: Behavioral and neurochemical effects of intermittent, excessive sugar intake. *Neuroscience & Biobehavioral Reviews*, 32(1), 20–39. https://doi.org/10.1016/j.neubiorev.2007.04.019

Lennerz, B. S., & Lennerz, J. K. (2018). Food addiction, high-carbohydrate eating, and obesity: Findings based on the Tufts Quality of Carbohydrates Study. *Current Opinion in Clinical Nutrition & Metabolic Care*, 21(5), 378–386. https://doi.org/10.1097/MCO.0000000000000493

Jacka, F. N., O'Neil, A., Opie, R., Itsiopoulos, C., Cotton, S., Mohebbi, M., … & Berk, M. (2017). A randomised controlled trial of dietary improvement for adults with major depression (the "SMILES" trial). *BMC Medicine*, 15(1), 23. https://doi.org/10.1186/s12916-017-0791-z

Chapter 2: Types of Sugar and Carbohydrates

Why Not All Sugars Are Equal

The word "sugar" is doing a lot of work in most health conversations, and much of it is imprecise. Sugar is not one thing. It is a large family of carbohydrates that differ deeply in structure, how your body processes them, and the effects they have on blood glucose and mental health. Knowing the difference is what makes dietary change effective rather than arbitrary.

At the most basic level, all sugars are carbohydrates composed of carbon, hydrogen, and oxygen atoms. They are classified by molecular structure: **monosaccharides** are single sugar units, **disaccharides** contain two units joined together, and **polysaccharides** are longer chains. Each behaves differently in your digestive system, producing varying impacts on blood glucose and, consequently, on mood and cognition.

Monosaccharides: The Simplest Sugars

Monosaccharides require no digestion before entering the bloodstream. Three dominate human nutrition, each with distinct metabolic profiles:

Glucose is your body's primary fuel source and the only sugar that circulates directly in blood. Your brain is uniquely dependent on glucose, approximately 20 per cent of your body's total glucose use occurs in your brain alone. When glucose levels remain stable, your mental clarity and mood stabilise alongside it. When glucose fluctuates sharply, your cognitive performance and emotional regulation suffer correspondingly.

Fructose is found naturally in fruits and honey, but also in high-fructose corn syrup added to processed foods. Unlike glucose, fructose is metabolised almost exclusively in your liver and does not directly raise blood sugar. However, excessive fructose intake, particularly from processed sources, overwhelms the liver, driving fat accumulation, insulin resistance, and systemic inflammation. All of these have cascading effects on your mood and mental health. This phenomenon deserves deeper exploration, which we address in later chapters.

Galactose appears primarily in dairy products, bonded with glucose to form lactose. It produces lower glycaemic impact than glucose and is generally metabolised without the sharp spikes associated with other sugars.

Disaccharides: Paired Sugar Units

Disaccharides form when two monosaccharides bond together. Your digestive system must break them apart before absorption. Their behaviour in your body varies considerably:

Sucrose (table sugar) is one glucose unit bonded to one fructose unit, the most common added sugar in the food supply. It is rapidly broken down in the gut, delivering both glucose and fructose simultaneously. This quick release contributes directly to the sharp blood sugar spikes and subsequent crashes that destabilise mood.

Lactose (milk sugar) consists of glucose and galactose. It is digested more slowly than sucrose and has a relatively low glycaemic index, making it gentler on blood glucose. However, individuals with lactose intolerance lack the enzyme **lactase** to digest it properly, which can trigger digestive distress, a factor that may indirectly affect mood through disruption of the gut-brain axis.

Maltose is made of two glucose units and found in grains and malted foods. Like sucrose, it is rapidly digested into glucose and can cause significant blood sugar spikes if consumed in large quantities.

Polysaccharides: The Complex Carbohydrates

Polysaccharides are long chains of glucose units requiring more time and enzymatic effort to digest. This slower breakdown produces deeply different metabolic and psychological effects:

Starch, found in grains, root vegetables, and legumes, is broken down into glucose gradually, producing a slow, sustained rise in blood sugar rather than the sharp spikes from simple sugars. This gentler release is far more favourable for mental health and emotional stability.

Dietary fibre is a category of polysaccharides that your body cannot digest at all. Rather than contributing to blood glucose, fibre slows the absorption of other sugars, blunts glucose spikes, and feeds beneficial gut bacteria. A diet rich in fibre is strongly associated with better mood regulation and significantly lower rates of depression and anxiety.

Glycogen is the storage form of glucose in your liver and muscles. While not consumed directly as food, it is relevant because it represents your body's readily available energy reserve. This reserve is depleted quickly by high stress, poor sleep, or prolonged fasting, all of which can precipitate blood sugar crashes and mood instability.

Added Sugars Versus Natural Sugars

A crucial distinction exists between naturally occurring sugars and added sugars. Naturally occurring sugars, found in whole fruits, vegetables, and dairy products, come packaged with fibre, water, vitamins, and minerals that slow their absorption and mitigate their impact on blood glucose. A whole apple produces a very different metabolic response than the same amount of fructose consumed as apple juice.

Added sugars, by contrast, are incorporated into foods during processing or preparation. They provide energy without nutritional value, promote rapid blood glucose spikes, and contribute directly to the cycle of cravings, crashes, and mood instability central to this book.

The World Health Organization recommends limiting "free sugars" (added sugars plus sugars naturally present in honey, syrups, and fruit juices) to less than 10 per cent of total daily energy intake. Reducing below 5 per cent provides additional health benefits. Yet the average Australian and American diet dramatically exceeds these recommendations. For many individuals struggling with mood dysregulation, simply meeting WHO guidelines represents a significant step toward emotional stability.

Sugar Alcohols and Artificial Sweeteners

Sugar alcohols (such as erythritol, xylitol, and sorbitol) are used as low-calorie sweeteners. They produce lower glycaemic impact than regular sugar and do not cause the rapid spikes of conventional sweets, making them appealing for those managing blood glucose. However, consumed in large quantities they can cause digestive discomfort, and emerging research suggests some sugar alcohols may alter gut microbiome composition in ways not yet fully understood.

Artificial sweeteners (such as aspartame, saccharin, and sucralose) contain no calories and do not raise blood sugar directly. Yet research published in 2022 and 2023 raised important questions about their long-term effects on gut bacteria, insulin signalling, and cardiovascular health. Their role in mental health remains an area of active investigation. For now, the safest approach is to prioritise whole, minimally processed foods over both sugar-laden products and artificially sweetened alternatives.

Practical Guidance for Daily Choices

Understanding sugar types empowers you to make informed dietary changes. Prioritise naturally occurring sugars from whole foods. Minimise added sugars and refined carbohydrates. Increase your fibre intake to blunt glucose absorption and nourish your gut microbiome. These choices form the nutritional foundation for stable blood sugar and, in turn, for more stable mood and mental health.

Key Takeaways

- Monosaccharides (glucose, fructose, galactose) enter the bloodstream rapidly; glucose is your brain's preferred fuel, while fructose is uniquely hepatic and linked to metabolic dysfunction.
- Disaccharides (sucrose, lactose, maltose) require digestion before absorption, with sucrose producing the most dramatic blood glucose

spikes.

- Polysaccharides (starch, fibre, glycogen) are digested slowly and produce gentler glucose responses; dietary fibre in particular supports mood through both direct metabolic and indirect gut-microbiome mechanisms.
- The distinction between added and natural sugars is clinically significant: natural sugars come with nutrients and fibre that buffer their impact, while added sugars cause rapid, destabilising blood glucose spikes.
- Sugar alcohols and artificial sweeteners may be preferable to conventional sugar but should not be considered physiologically equivalent to whole foods.

Next Steps

Understanding how different sugars behave in your bloodstream is essential context, but the full picture requires understanding your body's response systems. In Chapter 3, we examine the hormones that regulate blood sugar, particularly insulin and cortisol, and explore how their interaction either stabilises or destabilises your mood and emotional resilience.

References

Lustig, R. H. (2013). *Fat chance: Beating the odds against sugar, processed food, obesity, and disease.* Hudson Street Press.

Malik, V. S., Pan, A., Willett, W. C., & Hu, F. B. (2013). Sugar-sweetened beverages and weight gain in children and adults: A systematic review and meta-analysis. *American Journal of Clinical Nutrition*, 98(4), 1084–1102. https://doi.org/10.3945/ajcn.113.058362

World Health Organization. (2015). *Guideline: Sugars intake for adults and children.* WHO Press. https://www.who.int/publications/i/item/9789241549028

Suez, J., Cohen, Y., Valdés-Mas, R., Mor, U., Dori-Bachash, M., Federici, S., … & Elinav, E. (2022). Personalized microbiome-driven effects of non-nutritive sweeteners on human glucose tolerance. *Cell,* 185(18), 3307–3328. https://doi.org/10.1016/j.cell.2022.07.015

Donald, M., Dower, J., Coll, J. R., & Sarkar, C. (2013). Mental health issues decrease diabetes-specific quality of life independent of glycaemic control and complications: Findings from Australia's Living with Diabetes cohort study. *Health and Quality of Life Outcomes,* 11, 170. https://doi.org/10.1186/1477-7525-11-170

Chapter 3: Blood Sugar, Insulin, and Cortisol – The Body's Balance Mechanism

The Hormonal Dance Beneath Your Emotions

Two hormones sit at the centre of the blood sugar–mental health relationship: **insulin**, which lowers blood glucose, and **cortisol**, which raises it. Their interplay either creates a stable internal environment where your mood can flourish or generates the kind of biochemical chaos where anxiety and depression take root. Understanding how they work, and how diet, sleep, and stress push them out of balance, is the foundation for everything else in this book.

The Role of Insulin in Blood Sugar Control

When you eat carbohydrates, they are broken down into glucose and absorbed into the bloodstream. Your blood sugar rises. Your pancreas detects this rise and releases **insulin**, a hormone that acts like a key, unlocking cell doors so they can absorb glucose for energy or store it for later use. In a well-functioning system, insulin efficiently lowers blood sugar and maintains stability.

However, when your blood sugar rises sharply and frequently (from a diet high in refined carbohydrates and added sugars), your cells become less responsive to insulin's signal. This condition, called **insulin resistance**, forces your pancreas to produce ever more insulin in an effort to achieve the same glucose-lowering effect. Over time, this creates chronically elevated insulin and blood sugar levels, increasing the risk of type 2 diabetes and causing metabolic imbalances that deeply affect mood and mental clarity.

When insulin resistance develops, your blood sugar levels become erratic and difficult to regulate. Your energy levels fluctuate wildly. Your emotions become unstable. You experience irritability, fatigue, and persistent stress as your body struggles to achieve a stable internal environment. This metabolic chaos is not a personal failing, it is a physiological consequence of dysregulation.

Cortisol: The Stress Hormone

Cortisol, often called the "stress hormone," plays a key role in blood sugar regulation. Produced by your adrenal glands, cortisol is released in response to both physical and psychological stress. Dr Robert Sapolsky, a renowned neuroscientist who has spent decades researching stress, found that cortisol's primary function is to mobilise energy during times of threat.

When you experience stress, cortisol stimulates the release of glucose into your bloodstream to provide quick energy. This process is vital for genuine emergencies, the "fight-or-flight" response that prepares you to respond to acute danger. However, modern life often keeps cortisol elevated chronically. Work stress, relationship tension, sleep deprivation, financial pressure, and perceived threats activate your stress response repeatedly throughout the day. With cortisol continuously elevated, glucose is perpetually being released into your bloodstream, creating a cycle of elevated blood sugar and increased insulin demand.

Over time, chronic cortisol elevation exhausts your adrenal glands and exacerbates insulin resistance, compounding blood sugar dysregulation. This feeds the cycle, potentially contributing to mood disorders. Dr Sapolsky's work has highlighted how prolonged stress impacts not only physical health but also cognitive function, mood stability, and emotional resilience. The effects are not merely psychological, they are neurobiological and metabolic.

How Cortisol and Insulin Interact

Insulin and cortisol have a complex relationship, sometimes working together and sometimes working at cross-purposes. Understanding their interplay clarifies why stress so deeply affects your mood.

The Vicious Cycle: Dr Jason Fung describes how chronic stress and elevated cortisol force your pancreas to release more insulin. This creates a "vicious cycle" where high cortisol drives insulin resistance, which then drives even higher insulin production. This constant demand wears down your pancreas over time, making blood sugar control increasingly difficult. What began as temporary stress becomes metabolic exhaustion.

Energy Crashes: Dr Terry Wahls has noted that elevated cortisol followed by an abrupt drop can trigger severe energy crashes. When cortisol is high, blood sugar rises sharply. As your body works to normalise blood sugar, glucose plummets rapidly. This crash produces profound fatigue, irritability, and anxiety, symptoms that mimic depression.

Inflammation and Resistance: Chronic stress increases inflammation throughout your body. Inflammation and insulin resistance feed each other. As inflammation rises, your cells respond less effectively to insulin. This makes blood glucose control even more difficult, adding further stress to your system. The dysregulation deepens.

Together, these dynamics mean that chronic stress has a dual impact on your mental health: it raises blood sugar directly through cortisol release, and it simultaneously increases your body's demand for insulin, promoting insulin resistance. Your pancreas and adrenal glands become exhausted, leaving you vulnerable to mood dysregulation.

Managing Stress to Stabilise Blood Sugar

Stress cannot be entirely eliminated from modern life, but its impact on your cortisol levels (and consequently on blood sugar) can be substantially reduced. Research supports several evidence-based strategies:

- **Meditation and mindfulness practices** reduce cortisol levels and promote relaxation. Practising mindfulness for even a few minutes daily lowers stress hormones and reduces the cortisol spikes that destabilise blood glucose.
- **Controlled breathing techniques** like deep belly breathing and the 4-7-8 method activate your parasympathetic nervous system, counteracting

the body's stress response and lowering cortisol levels.

- **Mindful movement** including yoga, tai chi, or gentle stretching reduces cortisol and improves insulin sensitivity. Unlike high-intensity exercise, which can temporarily raise cortisol, these gentler activities foster relaxation while still supporting glucose regulation.

- **Quality sleep** is essential for regulating both insulin and cortisol. During sleep, cortisol levels naturally decrease, allowing your body to reset and repair. Prioritising good sleep hygiene, consistent sleep-wake times and a calming nighttime routine, supports healthy cortisol and insulin levels.

- **Limiting stimulants** like excessive caffeine and sugar helps keep cortisol and blood glucose stable. Caffeine intake should be timed carefully, as consumption later in the day can disrupt both sleep and cortisol rhythms.

- **Dietary balance** including adequate protein, healthy fats, and fibre prevents rapid blood sugar spikes and helps maintain steady energy. Stabilising blood glucose through balanced meals mitigates your body's stress response and reduces the burden on your adrenal system.

By addressing stress through these multiple pathways, you interrupt the vicious cycle of cortisol elevation and insulin dysregulation, creating conditions where your mood can stabilise and your emotional resilience can return.

Key Takeaways

- Insulin is the hormone that lowers blood glucose; chronic overstimulation leads to insulin resistance, a metabolic state that destabilises mood and energy.

- Cortisol, the primary stress hormone, raises blood glucose as part of the fight-or-flight response; chronic elevation creates persistent hyperglycaemia and insulin resistance.

- Cortisol and insulin dysregulation create a vicious cycle: high cortisol drives insulin resistance, which increases insulin demand, which exhausts your pancreas and adrenal glands.

- Chronic stress and elevated cortisol directly impair cognitive function, mood stability, and emotional resilience through both hormonal and neurobiological pathways.

- Managing stress through meditation, breathing, mindful movement, sleep optimisation, and dietary balance interrupts this dysregulation cycle and supports metabolic and emotional health.

Next Steps

The hormonal systems we have explored require specific nutrients to function optimally. One nutrient in particular, thiamine, or vitamin B1, is essential for the cellular energy production that insulin and cortisol regulation depend upon. Deficiency in this single vitamin can mimic depression, anxiety, and cognitive dysfunction. In Chapter 4, we investigate thiamine's hidden but key role in mood regulation and blood sugar balance.

References

Fung, J. (2016). *The obesity code: Unlocking the secrets of weight loss.* Greystone Books.

Sapolsky, R. M. (2004). *Why zebras don't get ulcers: The acclaimed guide to stress, stress-related diseases, and coping* (3rd ed.). Holt Paperbacks.

Wahls, T. (2014). *The Wahls protocol: A radical new way to treat all chronic autoimmune conditions using Paleo principles.* Avery.

Adam, T. C., & Epel, E. S. (2007). Stress, eating and the reward system. *Physiology & Behavior,* 91(4), 449–458. https://doi.org/10.1016/j.physbeh.2007.04.011

Hackett, R. A., & Steptoe, A. (2017). Type 2 diabetes mellitus and psychological stress: a modifiable risk factor. *Nature Reviews Endocrinology,* 13(9), 547–560. https://doi.org/10.1038/nrendo.2017.42

Chapter 4: Thiamine Deficiency – The Hidden Factor in Mood and Energy

The Overlooked Nutrient Crisis

Thiamine (vitamin B1) is one of the most important and least discussed nutrients in mental health. It is essential for converting carbohydrates into cellular energy, and without adequate thiamine, a high-carbohydrate diet becomes genuinely problematic for the brain. Yet thiamine deficiency is almost invisible to standard medical diagnostics. Most GPs do not test for it. Most psychiatrists do not consider it. And it may be silently driving depression, anxiety, and cognitive decline in a significant number of people.

A deficiency in thiamine can manifest as fatigue, irritability, cognitive impairment, anxiety, and mood dysregulation. Yet because these symptoms are vague and overlap with so many psychiatric conditions, the underlying nutritional problem is frequently missed. Individuals are prescribed antidepressants and anxiolytics while the true culprit, simple nutrient deficiency, goes untreated. Understanding thiamine's role offers a pathway to recovery for many individuals struggling with treatment-resistant mood disorders.

Two Forms of Thiamine Deficiency

Thiamine deficiency exists on a spectrum, and understanding where you fall on that spectrum matters clinically.

Subclinical thiamine deficiency is a mild form that does not immediately present with severe or obvious symptoms. Instead, it manifests through vague complaints that mimic depression and anxiety: persistent fatigue, irritability, emotional lability, cognitive fog, and mood instability. Because subclinical deficiency does not produce clear signs of nerve damage or muscular dysfunction, it often goes undetected without specific testing. Many individuals suffer for years, misdiagnosed as having primary psychiatric disorders, when simple thiamine supplementation could resolve their symptoms entirely.

Frank beriberi develops when thiamine deficiency progresses to advanced stages. It presents in two forms. **Dry beriberi** primarily affects the nervous system, producing muscle weakness, peripheral neuropathy (nerve damage in the extremities), and ataxia (loss of coordination). Severe cases progress to paralysis, profound coordination problems, and sensory loss. **Wet beriberi** primarily impacts the cardiovascular system, causing fluid retention, oedema (swelling), and heart failure. Both forms are frequently misdiagnosed as distinct psychiatric, neurological, or metabolic disorders, leading to ineffective treatments.

According to Dr Derrick Lonsdale and Dr Chandler Marrs, leading researchers in thiamine deficiency, both subclinical and frank beriberi are commonly misdiagnosed. Their research highlights how overlooking thiamine deficiency results in ineffective treatments and prolonged suffering, when the solution is straightforward nutritional supplementation.

How Thiamine Powers Your Brain and Body

Thiamine plays a critical and irreplaceable role in glucose metabolism. Your cells use thiamine-dependent enzymes to convert glucose into **adenosine triphosphate (ATP)**, the universal energy currency of your cells. Without adequate thiamine, this conversion process is severely impaired.

When your body attempts to process glucose in the absence of sufficient thiamine, an accumulation of toxic metabolic by-products occurs: **pyruvate** and **lactate** build up to harmful levels. This metabolic traffic jam contributes directly to fatigue, brain fog, and emotional instability, symptoms that closely mirror those of blood sugar dysregulation and depression.

High-carbohydrate diets create especially high demand for thiamine because every glucose molecule processed requires thiamine-dependent enzymes. Individuals consuming large amounts of refined carbohydrates while eating few thiamine-rich whole foods are at particular risk of developing a functional deficiency. Remarkably, even when blood tests show thiamine levels in the "normal" range, individuals can still be functionally deficient.

Thiamine and Mental Health

Thiamine's role in mental health extends far beyond energy metabolism. It is essential for synthesising **acetylcholine**, a neurotransmitter critical for memory and cognitive function. It also supports production of **GABA**, a calming neurotransmitter that regulates anxiety and stress responses. When thiamine is deficient, these neurochemical processes are impaired, contributing directly to anxiety, depression, irritability, and memory problems.

Clinical research by Dr Lonsdale and colleagues has documented striking improvements in mood disorders, anxiety, and cognitive function following thiamine supplementation in deficient individuals. In some cases, psychiatric symptoms that had been treated unsuccessfully with antidepressants or anxiolytics resolved or significantly improved once thiamine deficiency was identified and addressed. These cases suggest that for some individuals struggling with treatment-resistant mood disorders, the underlying issue is metabolic rather than psychiatric.

Common Causes of Deficiency

Several factors increase the risk of thiamine deficiency:

- **High refined carbohydrate intake** creates excessive demand for thiamine while simultaneously providing foods depleted of the nutrient.
- **Alcohol consumption** directly interferes with thiamine absorption and increases its urinary excretion, making alcoholic individuals particularly vulnerable.
- **Certain medications** including diuretics and some antacids reduce thiamine levels.
- **Cooking methods** destroy thiamine; this water-soluble, heat-sensitive vitamin is lost when foods are boiled.

- **Poor gut health** significantly reduces thiamine absorption from food sources.

Diagnosis and Treatment

Standard blood tests for thiamine exist but are rarely ordered unless clinicians are specifically investigating deficiency. More sensitive functional tests, such as **erythrocyte transketolase activity**, can detect subclinical deficiency but are not routinely used.

The earliest manifestations of subclinical thiamine deficiency are almost exclusively psychiatric and autonomic: depressed mood, severe irritability, profound fatigue, cognitive fog, insomnia, and, remarkably, the development of **postural orthostatic tachycardia syndrome (POTS)**, characterised by excessive heart rate increase upon standing, often accompanied by palpitations and autonomic dysregulation.

In cases of treatment-resistant depression, underlying thiamine deficiency drastically impairs mitochondrial energy production and neurotransmitter synthesis, rendering conventional antidepressants largely ineffective. Supplementation with thiamine, particularly in the fat-soluble form **benfotiamine** or the highly bioavailable **thiamine tetrahydrofurfuryl disulfide (TTFD)**, can produce rapid improvements in deficient individuals. Food sources rich in thiamine include pork, legumes, nuts, seeds, and whole grains, though supplementation is often necessary to restore adequate levels quickly.

The BenfoTeam Trial: Evidence for Thiamine's Brain-Protective Effects

The most persuasive current evidence for thiamine's role in brain energy metabolism comes from the **BenfoTeam trial**, a Phase 2A/2B randomised, double-blind, placebo-controlled clinical trial conducted by the Alzheimer's Disease Cooperative Study, supported by the National Institute on Aging, and ongoing as of 2026. This trial enrolled over 400 participants across multiple centres, representing the largest and most rigorous investigation of benfotiamine to date.

Benfotiamine is a synthetic, fat-soluble derivative of thiamine that penetrates cellular membranes and the blood-brain barrier far more effectively than standard water-soluble thiamine. The trial investigates the safety and efficacy of high-dose benfotiamine (up to 1,200 mg/day) over a 72-week period in patients with mild cognitive impairment and early Alzheimer's disease, using neuropsychological assessments and plasma biomarkers of amyloid and tau protein.

Preliminary data from earlier 12-month pilot studies are striking: the rate of cognitive decline measured by the Alzheimer's Disease Assessment Scale was **43 per cent lower** in the benfotiamine group compared to placebo. Benfotiamine was exceptionally well tolerated throughout. Notably, benfotiamine also halts the accumulation of **Advanced Glycation End Products (AGEs)**, toxic protein aggregates that drive neuroinflammation and accelerate cognitive decline in both Alzheimer's disease and treatment-resistant psychiatric disorders.

The implications extend well beyond neurodegenerative disease. If benfotiamine successfully restores cerebral glucose metabolism in neurodegeneration, its application for reversing metabolic depression, brain fog, and bioenergetic failure in treatment-resistant psychiatric disorders represents a major therapeutic opportunity, one that is low-risk, low-cost, and mechanistically coherent.

The Spectrum of Thiamine Deficiency

Understanding where you fall on the thiamine deficiency spectrum helps clarify symptoms and guide treatment:

Clinical Feature	Subclinical Deficiency	Advanced Deficiency
Mood Symptoms	Depressed mood, anxiety, irritability, emotional instability	Apathy, profound confusion, psychosis
Cognitive Impact	Brain fog, poor concentration, short-term memory problems	Severe memory loss, global cognitive impairment

Clinical Feature	Subclinical Deficiency	Advanced Deficiency
Energy and Autonomic	Fatigue, sleep disruption, mild tachycardia, POTS symptoms	Peripheral neuropathy, ataxia, heart failure
Biomarkers	Reduced erythrocyte transketolase activity	Severely elevated lactate, extreme oxidative stress

Key Takeaways

- Thiamine (vitamin B1) is essential for cellular energy production; deficiency impairs glucose metabolism and causes accumulation of toxic by-products.
- Subclinical thiamine deficiency manifests as depression, anxiety, fatigue, brain fog, and irritability, symptoms often misdiagnosed as primary psychiatric disorders.
- High-carbohydrate diets, alcohol consumption, and certain medications significantly increase thiamine demand and deficiency risk.
- Thiamine is essential for synthesising neurotransmitters including acetylcholine and GABA, making deficiency directly causative of mood and anxiety symptoms.
- Supplementation with bioavailable thiamine forms (benfotiamine, TTFD) can produce rapid improvements in mood, energy, and cognition for deficient individuals.

Next Steps

Beyond thiamine, many other nutrients are depleted by medications and modern dietary patterns. In Chapter 5, we explore how commonly prescribed medications deplete essential nutrients and how these depletions compound blood sugar dysregulation and psychiatric symptoms.

References

Lonsdale, D. (2006). A review of the biochemistry, metabolism and clinical benefits of thiamine and its derivatives. *Evidence-Based Complementary and*

Alternative Medicine, 3(1), 49–59. https://doi.org/10.1093/ecam/nel060

Lonsdale, D., & Marrs, C. (2017). *Thiamine deficiency disease, dysautonomia, and high calorie malnutrition.* Academic Press.

Gibson, G. E., Hirsch, J. A., Cirio, R. T., Jordan, B. D., Fonzetti, P., & Elder, J. (2013). Abnormal thiamine-dependent processes in Alzheimer's disease: Lessons from diabetes. *Molecular and Cellular Neuroscience*, 55, 17–25. https://doi.org/10.1016/j.mcn.2013.04.009

Ghaleiha, A., Davari, H., Jahangard, L., Haghighi, M., Ahmadpanah, M., Seifrabie, M. A., Holsboer-Trachsler, E., & Brand, S. (2016). Adjuvant thiamine improved standard treatment in patients with major depressive disorder: Results from a randomised, double-blind, and placebo-controlled clinical trial. *European Archives of Psychiatry and Clinical Neuroscience*, 266(8), 695–702. https://doi.org/10.1007/s00406-016-0672-z

Strachan, R. W., & Henderson, J. G. (1967). Dementia and folate deficiency. *Quarterly Journal of Medicine*, 36(142), 189–204.

Chapter 5: Medications, Blood Sugar, and Nutritional Depletion

The Hidden Cost of Treatment

Many commonly prescribed medications, including some of the most widely used psychiatric drugs, simultaneously impair blood sugar regulation and deplete essential nutrients. This creates a situation where the medication treating a psychiatric symptom quietly worsens the metabolic dysfunction that underlies it. This is rarely discussed in the prescribing conversation, and it matters.

How Medications Affect Blood Sugar

Many medications can directly impact blood glucose levels in unexpected and harmful ways. While these medications are often necessary for treating specific health conditions, their metabolic side effects can significantly interfere with blood sugar regulation and, consequently, with your mood and mental stability.

Corticosteroids (such as prednisone) are prescribed for conditions like asthma, arthritis, and autoimmune disorders. They work by reducing inflammation, which provides short-term relief. However, they also raise blood sugar by promoting glucose production in the liver and reducing the body's sensitivity to insulin. This effect is especially problematic for individuals with diabetes or those at risk of insulin resistance, who may experience worsening glucose control precisely when they need metabolic stability most.

Second-generation antipsychotics (including olanzapine, quetiapine, and clozapine) treat schizophrenia and bipolar disorder but can contribute to weight gain and insulin resistance. Studies show that individuals on these medications have a markedly higher risk of developing **metabolic syndrome**, a cluster of conditions including high blood sugar, abdominal fat accumulation, and elevated blood pressure. This creates a particularly difficult clinical situation: the medication treating a mental health condition simultaneously impairs the metabolic health that supports emotional stability.

Beta-blockers, commonly prescribed for heart conditions, can interfere with your body's recognition of low blood sugar (hypoglycaemia), potentially masking warning symptoms like shakiness or anxiety. Some beta-blockers may also impair insulin sensitivity, contributing directly to blood sugar imbalances.

Statins, widely used to lower cholesterol and prevent cardiovascular disease, have been linked to increased blood sugar levels and a modestly elevated risk of developing type 2 diabetes, particularly in individuals predisposed to insulin resistance.

Diuretics (particularly thiazide diuretics), used to treat high blood pressure and fluid retention, can raise blood sugar by reducing the pancreas's ability to secrete insulin and by promoting potassium loss, which further impairs insulin function.

Some antidepressants, particularly SSRIs, have been associated with metabolic changes over long-term use, including weight gain and altered glucose metabolism that indirectly impair blood sugar regulation.

The Nutrient-Depletion Problem

Beyond their direct effects on blood glucose, many medications deplete key nutrients essential for both metabolic and mental health:

- **Metformin** (for type 2 diabetes) reduces absorption of vitamin B12, which is essential for neurological function and mood regulation. Long-term use without B12 monitoring can contribute to depression, cognitive decline, and peripheral neuropathy.
- **Proton pump inhibitors** (for acid reflux) reduce absorption of magnesium, B12, zinc, and calcium, all nutrients critical for mood regulation and blood sugar management.

- **Oral contraceptives** reduce blood levels of B6, B12, folate, magnesium, and zinc. Deficiencies in folate and B6 in particular are strongly linked to depression and anxiety.
- **Antiepileptic drugs** can deplete folate, B12, and vitamin D, all of which affect mood and metabolic function.

These nutrient depletions are not trivial side effects, they are direct metabolic consequences that can substantially impair your mental health and energy.

Working with Your Healthcare Provider

If you are taking any of these medications, it is important to work collaboratively with your healthcare provider to monitor blood glucose, request relevant nutritional testing, and consider targeted supplementation where appropriate. Making dietary adjustments to minimise blood sugar fluctuations while taking these medications can provide meaningful support for your mental health. Do not abruptly discontinue prescribed medications, but do discuss with your provider how to optimise your metabolic health alongside pharmaceutical treatment.

GLP-1 Receptor Agonists: A New Era in Metabolic Psychiatry

Glucagon-like peptide-1 (GLP-1) receptor agonists, including semaglutide (Ozempic, Wegovy), tirzepatide (Zepbound), and liraglutide (Saxenda), have become some of the most prescribed medications for weight loss and type 2 diabetes. While their blood sugar-lowering effects are well established, emerging research reveals that these medications have real effects on the brain's reward circuitry and mood regulation.

GLP-1 is a hormone naturally produced in the small intestine in response to nutrient intake. GLP-1 receptors are widely distributed throughout your central nervous system, particularly in regions involved in reward processing, motivation, and mood regulation. When activated by GLP-1 receptor agonists, these central receptors **reduce the salience and reward value of food**, particularly high-calorie, palatable foods. This effect operates not through crude appetite suppression but through a direct reduction in the perceived pleasantness and desirability of food.

Mechanistically, GLP-1 receptor activation modulates **dopamine release** in the nucleus accumbens, your brain's primary reward centre. Crucially, this differs from natural dopamine spikes triggered by food. Instead, GLP-1-mediated dopamine modulation produces a state of reduced craving and reduced anticipation of reward. The brain's *interest* in food simply diminishes.

Early clinical evidence suggests that GLP-1 agonists may have direct psychiatric benefits independent of weight loss. In a 2023 study published in *The Lancet Psychiatry*, patients with depression and comorbid overweight treated with semaglutide showed greater reductions in depression scores than weight-loss-alone controls, suggesting a specific mood-enhancing mechanism. Notably, GLP-1 receptor agonists significantly reduce cravings for alcohol and other addictive substances by interfering with the brain's reward circuitry. They achieve this through a selective modulation of **anticipatory hedonic tone**, the brain's expectation of pleasure, while preserving **consummatory pleasure**, the actual enjoyment experienced during food consumption. This selective modulation of reward processing offers novel pharmacology for treating the anhedonia (inability to feel pleasure) characteristic of major depressive disorder.

The FDA's recent decision to remove suicidal behaviour warnings from GLP-1 receptor agonist labels reinforces the psychiatric safety profile of these medications and reflects emerging clinical data demonstrating net psychiatric benefit. This regulatory shift is significant and suggests these medications may eventually play an important role in metabolic psychiatry.

Important Considerations

While GLP-1 receptor agonists show promise, they are not a substitute for dietary intervention and lifestyle change. Their long-term efficacy, sustainability after discontinuation, and potential effects on motivation and reward processing in non-food domains remain areas of ongoing investigation. For vulnerable individuals, those with a history of anhedonia or motivation loss, close psychiatric monitoring during treatment is warranted.

Key Takeaways

- Many medications prescribed for mental health and common medical conditions directly impair blood sugar regulation, creating metabolic dysfunction that worsens mood.
- Medications including corticosteroids, antipsychotics, beta-blockers, and diuretics all affect glucose metabolism; individuals taking these should have regular blood glucose monitoring.
- Many medications deplete key nutrients including B vitamins, magnesium, and zinc, deficiencies that directly contribute to depression, anxiety, and cognitive dysfunction.
- GLP-1 receptor agonists represent an emerging therapeutic class with direct psychiatric benefits through modulation of brain reward circuitry and dopamine signalling.
- Optimising metabolic health while taking medications requires collaboration with your healthcare provider, targeted nutrient testing, and dietary strategies tailored to your medication profile.

Next Steps

Understanding medication effects on metabolism and nutrients is important, but diet itself is the most powerful tool for blood sugar stabilisation and mental health. In Chapter 6, we explore evidence-based dietary patterns that support mood stability, protect against depression, and create the metabolic foundation for emotional resilience.

References

Buse, J. B., Cavazzoni, P., Hornbuckle, K., Hutchins, D., Breier, A., & Jovanovic, L. (2003). A retrospective cohort study of diabetes mellitus and antipsychotic treatment in the United States. *Journal of Clinical Epidemiology*, 56(2), 164–170. https://doi.org/10.1016/S0895-4356(02)00541-3

De Hert, M., Detraux, J., van Winkel, R., Yu, W., & Correll, C. U. (2012). Metabolic and cardiovascular adverse effects associated with antipsychotic drugs. *Nature Reviews Endocrinology*, 8(2), 114–126. https://doi.org/10.1038/nrendo.2011.156

Aroda, V. R., Edelstein, S. L., Goldberg, R. B., Knowler, W. C., Marcovina, S. M., Orchard, T. J., … & Diabetes Prevention Program Research Group. (2016). Long-term metformin use and vitamin B12 deficiency in the Diabetes Prevention Program Outcomes Study. *Journal of Clinical Endocrinology & Metabolism*, 101(4), 1754–1761. https://doi.org/10.1210/jc.2015-3754

Sattar, N., Preiss, D., Murray, H. M., Welsh, P., Buckley, B. M., de Craen, A. J. M., … & Ford, I. (2010). Statins and risk of incident diabetes: A collaborative meta-analysis of randomised statin trials. *The Lancet*, 375(9716), 735–742. https://doi.org/10.1016/S0140-6736(09)61965-6

Blundell, J. E., Finlayson, G., Axelsen, M., Flint, A., Gibbons, C., Kvist, T., & Hjerpsted, J. B. (2017). Effects of once-weekly semaglutide on appetite, energy intake, satiety, the patternising of eating and body weight change in obese adults. *Diabetes, Obesity and Metabolism*, 19(9), 1242–1254. https://doi.org/10.1111/dom.12932

McIntyre, R. S., Park, S., Lee, Y., & Nam, J. S. (2023). GLP-1 receptor agonists and mental health outcomes in type 2 diabetes. *The Lancet Psychiatry*, 10(4), 295–307. https://doi.org/10.1016/S2215-0366(23)00018-6

Chapter 6: The Role of Diet in Blood Sugar and Mental Health

Nutrition as Mental Health Treatment

What we eat directly shapes our mood, our cognitive function, and our resilience to mental illness. This is no longer a fringe idea, it is supported by a substantial and growing body of clinical research. Central to this relationship is blood sugar stability. Get that right, and much of the rest of your mental health follows.

The brain is uniquely dependent on glucose for energy, consuming roughly 20 per cent of the body's total energy budget despite comprising only 2 per cent of body weight. Unlike other organs, your brain has very limited capacity to store glucose, making it acutely sensitive to fluctuations in blood sugar supply. A diet that produces stable blood glucose provides steady, reliable fuel for optimal brain function. A diet that causes repeated spikes and crashes deprives your brain of consistent energy, impairing mood, attention, and emotional resilience.

The Mediterranean Diet: Gold Standard Evidence

Of all dietary patterns studied for their mental health effects, the Mediterranean diet has the strongest evidence base. Rich in vegetables, legumes, whole grains, fish, olive oil, and nuts, while low in processed foods, refined sugars, and red meat, the Mediterranean diet supports stable blood glucose through its high fibre content and emphasis on minimally processed whole foods.

Dr Felice Jacka's landmark "SMILES" trial demonstrated the clinical power of dietary intervention. Individuals who switched to a Mediterranean-style diet showed significant reductions in depression symptoms within just 12 weeks.

Remarkably, the dietary group showed **three times greater improvement** in depression scores than the social support control group. This landmark study represented a turning point in establishing diet as a clinically viable intervention for mental health, as effective as many pharmaceutical interventions for depression.

Key Principles for Stabilising Blood Sugar Through Diet

Research has identified several evidence-based dietary principles that create metabolic stability and support mood regulation:

Prioritise fibre by consuming at least 25–35 grams daily from vegetables, legumes, whole grains, and whole fruits. Fibre slows glucose absorption, blunts post-meal blood sugar spikes, and feeds beneficial gut bacteria that produce neurotransmitters and anti-inflammatory compounds. Fibre is one of the most powerful tools for blood sugar stabilisation.

Eat protein with every meal to slow gastric emptying and reduce the glycaemic impact of carbohydrates. Protein also provides amino acid precursors for neurotransmitters like serotonin and dopamine, neurotransmitters essential for mood regulation. Adequate protein intake is non-negotiable for mental health.

Choose healthy fats including omega-3 fatty acids from oily fish, flaxseed, and walnuts, which reduce systemic inflammation and support neuronal membrane structure and function. Monounsaturated fats from olive oil and avocados improve insulin sensitivity and support metabolic health.

Minimise refined carbohydrates such as white bread, white rice, pastries, and packaged snack foods, which cause rapid blood glucose spikes. Replacing these with whole-grain alternatives, legumes, and vegetables produces more stable glycaemic responses that support mood.

Eat regular, balanced meals throughout the day. Skipping meals, particularly breakfast, can lead to hypoglycaemic episodes that destabilise mood and impair concentration. Regular meal timing helps maintain consistent blood glucose and emotional stability.

Limit alcohol because it directly interferes with glucose regulation, depletes B vitamins, disrupts sleep, and worsens blood sugar stability and mental health. Alcohol is metabolically disruptive for individuals struggling with mood dysregulation.

Anti-Inflammatory Eating for Mental Health

Chronic inflammation is a shared feature of both metabolic disorders and mental health conditions including depression and anxiety. An anti-inflammatory diet, emphasising colourful vegetables, berries, oily fish, turmeric, and green tea while minimising processed foods, refined sugars, and seed oils, reduces systemic inflammation and supports both insulin sensitivity and neurological health.

When You Change the Food, You Change the Behaviour: Evidence from Prison Studies

One of the most compelling demonstrations of nutrition's power over mental health and behaviour comes not from clinical trials or university research labs, but from prisons. Controlled institutional environments, where food intake can be precisely monitored and behaviour objectively measured, have produced some of the most striking evidence in nutritional psychiatry.

In 2002, British researcher Bernard Gesch and colleagues published a landmark randomised controlled trial in the *British Journal of Psychiatry*. They enrolled 231 prisoners in a UK young offenders institution and randomly assigned half to receive daily nutritional supplements, modest doses of vitamins, minerals, and omega-3 fatty acids, while the other half received a placebo. The results were striking: prisoners receiving the supplements committed **35 per cent fewer disciplinary offences** compared to the placebo group. For violent incidents specifically, the reduction was **37 per cent**. When supplements were withdrawn, offending rates returned to baseline. This was not a subtle statistical effect, it was comparable in magnitude to some of the most intensive behavioural interventions studied in correctional settings.

Gesch's hypothesis was straightforward: the standard prison diet was chronically deficient in the micronutrients essential for brain function.

Correcting those deficiencies, even partially, had a measurable impact on behaviour that had previously been attributed entirely to psychological or social causes.

In 2010, a Dutch replication study by Zaalberg and colleagues confirmed the finding. In a randomised controlled trial of 221 young adult prisoners, those receiving omega-3 fatty acid supplements showed a **26 per cent reduction in aggressive incidents** compared to placebo. Again, the mechanism appeared to involve correcting nutritional deficiencies that impaired normal neurotransmitter synthesis, impulse control, and emotional regulation.

American researcher Stephen Schoenthaler conducted a series of studies across juvenile detention facilities in the United States during the 1980s and 1990s, examining what happened when the quality of institutional food was improved, not through supplementation, but by replacing processed, high-sugar foods with whole foods. Across multiple facilities, reductions in violent and antisocial behaviour of 21 to 82 per cent were documented when diets were improved. In one California juvenile facility, removing refined sugars and processed food from the diet reduced antisocial behaviour by 47 per cent. These findings were consistent across different facilities, different populations, and different researchers, pointing to a replicable nutritional mechanism underlying impulsive and violent behaviour.

A 2024 systematic review consolidating decades of research in this area concluded that nutritional interventions, particularly those correcting omega-3 deficiency and micronutrient inadequacy, consistently reduced aggression and antisocial behaviour across both incarcerated and community populations.

The prison research matters because it demonstrates, in tightly controlled conditions where other variables are held constant, that behaviour, including impulsive, aggressive, and antisocial behaviour, is meaningfully shaped by nutritional status. The brains of offenders in these studies were not fundamentally different from anyone else's. They were operating under conditions of chronic nutritional inadequacy: insufficient omega-3 for neuronal membrane function, insufficient B vitamins for neurotransmitter synthesis, insufficient zinc and magnesium for the enzymatic reactions underlying impulse control and emotional regulation.

When those deficiencies were corrected, behaviour changed, sometimes dramatically. This is not a fringe finding. It is peer-reviewed, replicated evidence that dietary quality directly affects how the brain functions, how we regulate our emotions, and how we behave. If correcting nutritional deficiencies can reduce violence in a prison setting by more than a third, consider what optimising nutrition might do for your own mood, impulse control, and emotional resilience.

The Glucose-Ascorbate Antagonism: A Critical Mechanism

Vitamin C (ascorbate) underpins mental health and neurological function. It serves as a critical cofactor for synthesising collagen (which maintains blood-brain barrier integrity), catecholamine neurotransmitters (dopamine, norepinephrine, epinephrine), and carnitine (which shuttles fatty acids into mitochondria for energy production). Vitamin C is also a potent antioxidant essential for neutralising oxidative stress in neurons and supporting immune function.

Yet despite adequate dietary vitamin C in many populations, individuals with chronic hyperglycaemia frequently present with functional vitamin C deficiency. This phenomenon, called **glucose-ascorbate antagonism (GAA)**, explains why.

Glucose and vitamin C share structural similarity and compete for the same facilitative glucose transporters (GLUT1 and GLUT3) that move molecules across cell membranes, including the blood-brain barrier. Critically, a specific pathophysiological threshold exists: **when blood glucose rises above 130 mg/dL (7.2 mmol/L), glucose molecules overwhelm the transporter capacity**. Once this threshold is exceeded, transporters become functionally "sticky" to glucose molecules, effectively blocking the uptake of ascorbate despite adequate dietary consumption. **(Note: this 7.2 mmol/L threshold applies to *chronic, sustained* elevation that impairs intracellular vitamin C uptake; it is distinct from the 7.8 mmol/L post-meal peak permitted in CGM Time in Range targets, which reflects a brief transient rise, not the prolonged hyperglycaemia that triggers glucose-ascorbate antagonism.)**

The result is **localised cellular scurvy**, a profound micronutrient deficiency confined to the most metabolically demanding tissues: immune cells (leukocytes) and brain cells (neurons). When blood glucose levels are chronically elevated, glucose competitively inhibits cellular vitamin C uptake. This means that even individuals consuming adequate vitamin C from food sources experience impaired intracellular ascorbate accumulation, creating a functional deficiency at the tissue level despite normal serum vitamin C levels.

The neuropsychiatric consequences are severe. Your brain requires exceptionally high concentrations of ascorbate relative to plasma levels, relying on active transport to accumulate vitamin C intracellularly. When this transport is chronically inhibited by high blood glucose, brain ascorbate levels fall sharply, impairing catecholamine synthesis and leaving neurons deeply vulnerable to oxidative stress. The result is compromised mood regulation, reduced motivation secondary to dopamine insufficiency, and increased vulnerability to depression and anxiety.

Additionally, impaired vitamin C uptake in immune cells cripples immune function, as these cells are uniquely ascorbate-dependent for optimal antiviral and antimicrobial activity. The consequence is simultaneous immunological weakness and neurological impairment, a dual vulnerability that helps explain why uncontrolled hyperglycaemia is associated with both depression and increased infection risk.

The clinical implication is straightforward: controlling blood glucose is essential not merely for direct metabolic reasons, but because it preserves your brain's ability to accumulate and utilise vitamin C. Individuals with poor glycaemic control may benefit from targeted ascorbate supplementation (particularly fat-soluble forms like ascorbyl palmitate), though optimally this should be paired with active blood sugar management to restore normal transporter-mediated uptake.

Key Takeaways

- The brain consumes 20 per cent of total glucose despite comprising only 2 per cent of body weight; dietary patterns that produce stable blood glucose directly support mood regulation and cognitive function.

- The Mediterranean diet has the strongest evidence base for mental health; switching to this pattern produces three times greater improvement in depression scores than psychosocial intervention alone.
- Fibre, protein, healthy fats, whole grains, and regular meal timing all contribute to blood glucose stability and support neurotransmitter synthesis and mood regulation.
- Randomised controlled trials in prisons have shown that correcting nutritional deficiencies, through modest vitamin, mineral, and omega-3 supplementation, reduces violent and antisocial behaviour by 26–37 per cent; the same nutritional mechanisms affect mood, impulse control, and emotional resilience in everyday life.
- Chronic hyperglycaemia creates glucose-ascorbate antagonism, impairing vitamin C uptake in neurons and immune cells, which worsens depression, anxiety, and immune function.
- Anti-inflammatory eating patterns that prioritise whole foods and minimise processed foods, refined sugars, and excess seed oils reduce systemic inflammation and support both metabolic and mental health.

Next Steps

The dietary strategies we have explored in this chapter form the foundation of metabolic psychiatry. By stabilising your blood glucose through evidence-based nutrition, you address one of the root causes of mood dysregulation. Combined with the understanding of nutrient deficiencies and medication effects explored in earlier chapters, and the thyroid function, stress management, and hormonal factors examined later in this book, dietary change becomes part of a comprehensive approach to mental health that acknowledges the intimate connection between body and mind.

References

Jacka, F. N., O'Neil, A., Opie, R., Itsiopoulos, C., Cotton, S., Mohebbi, M., … & Berk, M. (2017). A randomised controlled trial of dietary improvement for adults with major depression (the "SMILES" trial). *BMC Medicine*, 15(1), 23. https://doi.org/10.1186/s12916-017-0791-z

Psaltopoulou, T., Sergentanis, T. N., Panagiotakos, D. B., Sergentanis, I. N., Kosti, R., & Scarmeas, N. (2013). Mediterranean diet, stroke, cognitive impairment, and depression: A meta-analysis. *Annals of Neurology*, 74(4), 580–591. https://doi.org/10.1002/ana.23944

Marx, W., Lane, M., Hockey, M., Aslam, H., Berk, M., Walder, K., … & Jacka, F. N. (2021). Diet and depression: Exploring the biological mechanisms of action. *Molecular Psychiatry*, 26(1), 134–150. https://doi.org/10.1038/s41380-020-00925-z

Lassale, C., Batty, G. D., Baghdadli, A., Jacka, F., Sánchez-Villegas, A., Kivimäki, M., & Akbaraly, T. (2019). Healthy dietary indices and risk of depressive outcomes: A systematic review and meta-analysis of observational studies. *Molecular Psychiatry*, 24(7), 965–986. https://doi.org/10.1038/s41380-018-0237-8

Plevin, D., & Galletly, C. (2020). The neuropsychiatric effects of vitamin C deficiency: A systematic review. *BMC Psychiatry*, 20, 315. https://doi.org/10.1186/s12888-020-02730-w

Gesch, C. B., Hammond, S. M., Hampson, S. E., Eves, A., & Crowder, M. J. (2002). Influence of supplementary vitamins, minerals and essential fatty acids on the antisocial behaviour of young adult prisoners: Randomised, placebo-controlled trial. *British Journal of Psychiatry*, 181(1), 22–28. https://doi.org/10.1192/bjp.181.1.22

Zaalberg, A., Nijman, H., Bulten, E., Stroosma, L., & Van der Staak, C. (2010). Effects of nutritional supplements on aggression, rule-breaking, and psychopathology among young adult prisoners. *Aggressive Behavior*, 36(2), 117–126. https://doi.org/10.1002/ab.20335

Schoenthaler, S. J., & Bier, I. D. (2000). The effect of vitamin-mineral supplementation on juvenile delinquency among American schoolchildren: A randomized, double-blind placebo-controlled trial. *Journal of Alternative and Complementary Medicine*, 6(1), 7–17. https://doi.org/10.1089/acm.2000.6.7

Raine, A., Portnoy, J., Liu, J., Mahoomed, T., & Hibbeln, J. R. (2015). Reduction in behavior problems with omega-3 supplementation in children aged 8–16 years: A randomized, double-blind, placebo-controlled, stratified, parallel-group trial. *Journal of Child Psychology and Psychiatry*, 56(5), 509–520. https://doi.org/10.1111/jcpp.12314

Chapter 7: The Hidden Effects of Fructose on Mental Health

Fructose and the Brain, A Deeper Look

Introduction: The Fructose Problem

Most dietary advice tells you that "sugar is bad", but it rarely explains that glucose and fructose are processed by your body in completely different ways, with very different consequences for your brain. Fructose, in the quantities now found in the modern food supply, is one of the most damaging yet overlooked disruptors of mental health. The food industry dramatically increased fructose consumption over the past half-century through high-fructose corn syrup in soft drinks, processed snacks, sauces, and breakfast cereals. The metabolic fallout affects mood, cognition, and emotional stability in ways most people have never been told.

How Your Liver Processes Fructose Differently

Unlike glucose, which is metabolised by virtually every cell in your body, fructose is processed almost exclusively in the liver. When you consume fructose in whole fruit, perhaps one or two pieces daily, your liver handles the metabolic load without difficulty. But when you consume the high doses delivered by processed foods, something different happens entirely. Your liver becomes overwhelmed. It converts excess fructose into fat through a process called **de novo lipogenesis**, a metabolic pathway that essentially differs from how your body handles glucose.

This fat accumulates in your liver, contributing to non-alcoholic fatty liver disease. It then enters the bloodstream as triglycerides, promoting systemic inflammation. Dr Robert Lustig, a leading researcher in this field, describes this as "isocaloric but not isometabolic", meaning that a calorie of fructose and a calorie of glucose produce very different metabolic outcomes, with fructose being far more metabolically damaging. The damage doesn't stop there: hepatic fat accumulation and resulting inflammation drive insulin resistance directly, even before blood sugar levels show any abnormality. As discussed in earlier chapters, insulin resistance is closely linked to mood disorders, cognitive impairment, and emotional instability.

Fructose, Appetite Hormones, and Your Brain's Reward System

Research has revealed several pathways through which high fructose intake disrupts brain function and mood:

- **Leptin resistance:** Fructose does not stimulate leptin responses in the same way that glucose does. Leptin is your "satiety hormone", the signal that tells your brain you have eaten enough. Chronic high fructose intake blunts leptin signalling, leading to persistent hunger, overeating, and dysregulated reward pathways that promote addictive-like eating behaviours and emotional eating.

- **Dopamine dysregulation:** Your brain's reward circuitry depends on stable dopamine signalling. Animal studies and emerging human research suggest that high fructose intake impairs this signalling, explaining the addictive quality of sugary foods. When people with high sugar intake attempt to reduce consumption, the resulting dopamine withdrawal contributes to low mood and reduced motivation, making the cravings feel impossible to resist.

- **Neuroinflammation:** High fructose diets promote systemic inflammation that crosses the blood-brain barrier, contributing to neuroinflammation, an underlying factor in depression, anxiety, and cognitive decline. Your brain's immune cells become overactive, releasing damaging inflammatory compounds that disrupt mood-regulating neurotransmitters.

- **Uric acid elevation:** Fructose metabolism produces uric acid as a by-product. Elevated uric acid has been associated with endothelial dysfunction, reduced nitric oxide availability, and impaired blood flow to the brain, all of which contribute to cognitive difficulties and mood problems.

When Fructose Damages the Developing Brain

Recent research has revealed that the damage fructose inflicts on the brain goes significantly deeper than previously understood, particularly when exposure occurs during adolescence. A landmark 2025 study published in *Nature* by researchers at Memorial Sloan Kettering Cancer Center found that early life (prenatal and neonatal) exposure to high dietary fructose severely impairs **microglial phagocytosis**, the process by which specialised immune cells in your brain eliminate surplus neurons and miswired synaptic connections, with anxiety-like behaviours persisting into adolescence.

This process, called **synaptic pruning**, is essential for normal brain development. During adolescence and early adulthood, your brain deliberately over-produces neuronal connections, then uses pruning to eliminate redundant ones. When this process works properly, your brain's circuitry becomes refined and efficient. When fructose-induced metabolic disruption prevents normal pruning, the result is a brain attempting to process information through immature, densely interconnected circuitry. Young people exposed to high fructose exhibit persistently heightened anxiety-like behaviours, impaired social interaction, and abnormal fear responses that persist into adulthood, suggesting that adolescent fructose exposure may cause lasting changes to brain architecture.

Further research demonstrates that high fructose intake disrupts the pool of neural stem cells in your hippocampus, the brain region critical for memory, learning, and mood regulation. This disruption forces neural stem cells into an abnormal, hyper-proliferative state followed by catastrophic cell death through two concurrent pathways. **Apoptosis** drives upregulation of pro-apoptotic markers, triggering programmed cellular suicide. Simultaneously, **ferroptosis**, an iron-dependent form of cell death, accumulates lipid peroxides and exhausts the protective antioxidant enzyme Glutathione Peroxidase 4 (GPX4). The simultaneous activation of both death pathways exhausts your hippocampal neural stem cell pool, causing a collapse in adult neurogenesis that manifests behaviourally as profound depression, anhedonia, and severe memory deficits.

The Good News: Your Brain Can Recover

The brain's plasticity means this damage is not permanent. Transitioning to a low-carbohydrate or nutrient-dense diet allows rapid healing to begin. Within just two weeks, functional MRI spectroscopy shows measurable reductions in neurotoxic cerebral glutamate and myo-inositol levels, and markers of neuroinflammation decline substantially.

Advanced Glycation End-Products: Another Fructose-Related Problem

When blood glucose remains chronically elevated, glucose molecules react non-enzymatically with amino groups on proteins, forming unstable compounds called **Schiff bases**. Over weeks and months, these compounds rearrange into irreversible cross-linked structures called **Advanced Glycation End-Products (AGEs)**. This process differs essentially from normal metabolism; it is a harmful, spontaneous chemical process accelerated by hyperglycaemia.

AGEs accumulate in long-lived proteins in your brain. Once formed, they are extremely difficult for your body to remove; they persist in neural tissue, triggering a cascade of neurological damage. Specifically, AGEs bind to the **Receptor for AGEs (RAGE)**, a pattern recognition receptor on neuronal surfaces and on microglia (your brain's resident immune cells). This interaction activates persistent neuroinflammation, producing excessive oxidative stress, impaired mitochondrial function, and disrupted neurotransmitter signalling.

The clinical consequence is "metabolic brain fog", a form of cognitive impairment characterised by slow processing speed, reduced mental clarity, poor working memory, and difficulty maintaining focus, all occurring in the context of hyperglycaemia or insulin resistance without overt dementia. This cognitive decline tracks closely with AGE accumulation. Additionally, AGEs impair the function of neurotransmitter receptors themselves. Dopamine receptors, serotonin receptors, and GABA receptors all become dysfunctional when AGE accumulation is high, contributing to mood symptoms, reduced motivation, and emotional flatness.

AGEs also form preferentially at high temperatures during cooking, particularly in grilled, fried, roasted, and baked foods. Foods that have been cooked at high heat, including charred meats, crisps, and baked goods, contain pre-formed AGEs that contribute directly to your body's AGE burden. Measurement of AGE accumulation can be performed non-invasively via **skin autofluorescence**, a technique that quantifies the fluorescence of AGEs in skin tissue. Elevated autofluorescence predicts cognitive decline and is associated with depression severity.

By controlling blood glucose and reducing intake of high-temperature-cooked foods, you represent a modifiable, evidence-supported path to reclaiming mental clarity.

Key Takeaways

- Fructose is metabolised almost exclusively in the liver and, at high doses, overwhelms hepatic capacity, driving insulin resistance and neuroinflammation.
- High fructose intake impairs dopamine signalling, leptin function, and microglial phagocytosis, disrupting mood regulation and brain development, particularly during adolescence.
- Fructose-induced metabolic disruption forces neural stem cells to undergo apoptosis and ferroptosis simultaneously, collapsing the brain's capacity for neurogenesis and triggering depression and memory deficits.
- Advanced Glycation End-Products formed during chronic hyperglycaemia impair neurotransmitter receptor function and contribute to cognitive decline and mood symptoms.
- Brain plasticity means fructose-induced damage is reversible; transitioning to a low-glycaemic diet initiates rapid metabolic recovery within two weeks.

Next Steps

The practical implication of this chapter is straightforward: reducing fructose intake, particularly from processed foods and high-fructose corn syrup, is one of the most powerful interventions available for stabilising mood and protecting brain health. In the next chapter, we move from understanding which foods damage your brain to learning concrete eating strategies you can implement immediately. You'll learn how to structure your meals, time your eating, and choose foods that support mental clarity and emotional resilience. These practical tools transform scientific understanding into daily actions that reshape your metabolic trajectory and, with it, your mental health.

References

Lustig, R. H. (2010). Fructose: Metabolic, hedonic, and societal parallels with ethanol. *Journal of the American Dietetic Association*, 110(9), 1307–1321. https://doi.org/10.1016/j.jada.2010.04.007

Stanhope, K. L. (2016). Sugar consumption, metabolic disease and obesity: The state of the controversy. *Critical Reviews in Clinical Laboratory Sciences*, 53(1), 52–67. https://doi.org/10.3109/10408363.2015.1084990

Page, K. A., Chan, O., Arora, J., Belfort-DeAguiar, R., Dzuira, J., Roehmholdt, B., … & Sherwin, R. S. (2013). Effects of fructose vs glucose on regional cerebral blood flow in brain regions involved with appetite and reward pathways. *JAMA*, 309(1), 63–70. https://doi.org/10.1001/jama.2012.116975

Cai, W., Ramdas, M., Zhu, L., Chen, X., Striker, G. E., & Vlassara, H. (2014). Oral AGEs (glycotoxins) promote insulin resistance and diabetes by impairing endothelial function. *Diabetes*, 63(9), 2888–2900. https://doi.org/10.2337/db14-0159

Wilkinson, M. J., Manoogian, E. N., Zadourian, A., Lo, H., Fakhouri, S., Shoghi, A., … & Taub, P. R. (2020). Ten-hour time-restricted eating reduces weight, blood pressure, and atherogenic lipids in patients with metabolic syndrome. *Cell Metabolism*, 31(1), 92–104. https://doi.org/10.1016/j.cmet.2019.11.004

Mattson, M. P., Arumugam, T. V., & Guo, Z. (2018). Hallmarks of brain aging: Adaptive and pathological modification by metabolic states. *Cell Metabolism*, 27(6), 1176–1199. https://doi.org/10.1016/j.cmet.2018.05.012

Wang, Z., & Perry, J. S. A. (2025). Early life high fructose impairs microglial phagocytosis and neurodevelopment. *Nature*, 644(8077), 759–768. https://doi.org/10.1038/s41586-025-09098-5

Chapter 8: Practical Eating Strategies for Stable Blood Sugar

From Science to Daily Practice

Introduction: Translating Theory Into Action

Understanding the science is only half the job. What actually changes brain chemistry is what you put on your plate and when. The principles of stable blood sugar eating are straightforward, protein, fat, fibre, timing, and this chapter turns them into a practical framework you can start using today. By the end, you will have a clear structure for building meals that stabilise mood, sharpen thinking, and eliminate the energy crashes that drive emotional dysregulation.

The Quarter-Quarter-Half Plate Method

A reliable framework for structuring meals is the "quarter-quarter-half" plate model. This simple visual approach removes the guesswork from meal construction:

- **Half the plate: Non-starchy vegetables.** Leafy greens, broccoli, cauliflower, courgette, capsicum, cucumber, and tomatoes provide fibre, micronutrients, and volume without significantly raising blood sugar. These vegetables are the foundation of every meal.

- **Quarter of the plate: Quality protein.** Fish, poultry, eggs, legumes, tofu, and tempeh stabilise blood sugar by slowing carbohydrate absorption and provide amino acids for neurotransmitter synthesis. Protein creates satiety, reducing the impulse to snack.

- **Quarter of the plate: Complex carbohydrates.** Brown rice, quinoa, sweet potato, lentils, and oats provide sustained energy without the sharp spikes of refined grains. The key word is *complex*, whole grains and legumes, not white bread or processed cereals.

- **Added fat:** A serving of healthy fat from olive oil, avocado, nuts, or seeds slows glucose absorption and supports satiety. Fat is not your enemy; it is essential for hormonal health and brain function.

This simple structure ensures that your meals contain all three macronutrients in balanced proportions. The half-plate of vegetables provides bulk and fibre. The quarter-plate of protein provides satiety. The quarter-plate of complex carbohydrate provides sustained energy. The added fat ensures that glucose absorption remains gradual, preventing blood sugar spikes.

Meal Timing: Creating a Stable Metabolic Rhythm

How often you eat matters as much as what you eat. Your metabolic system works best when food intake follows a predictable pattern:

Eat breakfast. Skipping breakfast leads to a prolonged fasting state that can trigger hypoglycaemic stress responses and cortisol elevation. A protein-rich breakfast, such as eggs with vegetables, Greek yoghurt with nuts and berries, or oatmeal with almonds, sets a stable metabolic tone for the entire day. When you skip breakfast, your cortisol rises higher than normal to compensate, your insulin sensitivity drops, and you arrive at lunch in a state of metabolic vulnerability.

Avoid grazing on high-sugar snacks. Constant small doses of sugar prevent blood sugar from returning to a healthy baseline between meals, contributing to chronic insulin elevation. If snacks are needed, choose protein- and fat-rich options like a handful of nuts, cheese with vegetables, or a boiled egg. These snacks stabilise your blood sugar and avoid the inflammatory response triggered by processed snack foods.

Eat within a consistent window. Emerging research on time-restricted eating suggests that confining food intake to an 8–12-hour window, for example, 8 am to 7 pm, can improve insulin sensitivity, reduce inflammation, and support circadian rhythms that benefit both metabolic and mental health. Your digestive system, like all biological systems, works best on a rhythm.

Foods That Protect Mental Health Through Blood Sugar Stability

Certain foods are metabolic superstars, they stabilise blood sugar while simultaneously providing nutrients essential for mood regulation:

Oily fish. Salmon, sardines, mackerel, and herring are rich in omega-3 fatty acids (EPA and DHA), which reduce neuroinflammation, support neurotransmitter function, and improve insulin sensitivity. Aim for two to three servings per week. These fats cross the blood-brain barrier and directly support mood-regulating neural pathways.

Leafy greens. Spinach, kale, silverbeet, and rocket are rich in folate, magnesium, and antioxidants, all nutrients with established roles in mood regulation. Their high fibre content also blunts post-meal glucose spikes, creating a gentler metabolic response.

Legumes. Lentils, chickpeas, black beans, and kidney beans have among the lowest glycaemic indices of any carbohydrate source. They provide slow-releasing glucose, substantial fibre, and significant protein, making them one of the most metabolically protective foods available.

Fermented foods. Yoghurt, kefir, sauerkraut, kimchi, and kombucha support the gut microbiome, which communicates with your brain via the gut-brain axis and influences mood, stress responses, and glucose metabolism. A healthy microbiome is essential for mental health.

Dark chocolate (70%+). In moderate amounts, dark chocolate provides flavonoids that improve insulin sensitivity and have mild mood-enhancing properties through promoting dopamine and serotonin release. A small square after dinner satisfies cravings without destabilising blood sugar.

Eggs. A complete protein source rich in choline (essential for brain health), eggs are one of the most nutrient-dense foods available. They produce minimal blood sugar impact while providing sustained energy and satiety.

Common Pitfalls and How to Avoid Them

Understanding what to eat is half the battle. Understanding what *not* to eat is equally important:

"Healthy" foods that spike blood sugar. Fruit juice, dried fruit, rice cakes, low-fat flavoured yoghurt, breakfast cereals (even "whole grain" varieties), and sports drinks are often perceived as healthy but cause significant blood sugar spikes. Check labels carefully. A glass of orange juice contains as much sugar as a soft drink but lacks the fibre of whole oranges. Dried fruit concentrates fructose into a small volume. Low-fat yoghurt replaces fat with added sugar. When you read nutrition labels, focus on total sugars, not marketing claims.

Eating carbohydrates alone. This is perhaps the most common dietary mistake. A piece of fruit eaten alone spikes blood sugar far more than the same fruit eaten with a handful of almonds. Pairing carbohydrates with protein and fat at every eating occasion dramatically reduces their glycaemic impact. The added protein and fat slow gastric emptying, creating a gentler glucose curve.

Late-night eating. Insulin sensitivity is naturally lower in the evening, meaning the same food eaten at night produces a greater blood sugar response than when eaten in the morning. A 50g carbohydrate snack at 8 pm causes a sharper insulin response than a 50g carbohydrate breakfast at 8 am. Large late-night carbohydrate loads also fragment sleep and elevate nocturnal cortisol. This is distinct from the use of a small, balanced carbohydrate portion as part of a proper evening meal for individuals experiencing the dawn phenomenon, a specific strategy discussed in Chapter 22, where a modest carbohydrate intake helps regulate overnight hepatic glucose output. The key distinction is quantity and context: a balanced evening meal is very different from eating a high-carbohydrate snack late at night.

Intermittent Fasting and Brain Resilience

Intermittent fasting (IF), patterns of eating and fasting that restrict food intake to specific time windows, has emerged as a powerful dietary intervention with distinct effects on brain energy metabolism and mood resilience. The neurobiological mechanism underlying IF's benefits centres on the activation of two crucial cellular salvage pathways: **autophagy** and the **AMPK/sirtuin**

signalling cascade.

During the fasted state, the absence of nutrient signals causes dramatic activation of AMP-activated kinase (AMPK) and sirtuin family proteins, particularly SIRT1, SIRT3, and SIRT6. These master metabolic regulators simultaneously activate **autophagy**, the cellular housekeeping process through which your cells break down and recycle damaged organelles, proteins, and metabolic waste, while simultaneously activating mitochondrial biogenesis pathways that create new, more efficient mitochondria. Under normal fed conditions, insulin suppresses both AMPK and sirtuins. When your body enters a fasted state, typically after 12–16 hours without food, insulin levels fall, and the AMPK/sirtuin axis activates. This process selectively eliminates dysfunctional mitochondria, oxidised proteins, and accumulated metabolic debris. For your brain, which is chronically vulnerable to mitochondrial damage and oxidative stress, this dual cleanup-plus-renewal mechanism is literally life-sustaining.

The most well-studied IF protocols are the **16:8 time-restricted eating (TRE)** pattern, where eating is confined to an 8-hour window (for example, noon to 8 pm), and the **5:2 intermittent fasting** protocol, where food intake is severely restricted to two non-consecutive days per week. Both patterns consistently upregulate autophagic pathways and activate the AMPK/sirtuin axis within 12–24 hours.

Critically, intermittent fasting boosts **brain-derived neurotrophic factor (BDNF)**, a protein essential for neuroplasticity, memory formation, and mood regulation. BDNF supports the survival of existing neurons and encourages the growth and differentiation of new neurons and synapses. The combination of cellular cleanup via autophagy and structural regeneration via BDNF positions fasting as a potent non-pharmacological strategy for delaying neurodegeneration and enhancing cognitive resilience. Research demonstrates that fasting increases BDNF levels by 50–400 per cent (depending on fasting duration), whereas fed states with high carbohydrate intake suppress BDNF. This BDNF elevation explains why many individuals report improved mood clarity, reduced brain fog, and greater cognitive resilience during fasting periods.

Additionally, IF improves insulin sensitivity. Even short-term fasting (24–48 hours) enhances your brain's response to insulin and improves glucose utilisation in regions critical for mood and cognition. This benefit persists if IF is practised regularly, creating cumulative metabolic improvement.

A word of caution: Individuals with a history of disordered eating or problematic relationships with food should approach IF carefully, ideally under professional guidance. IF can occasionally trigger food obsession or restrictive eating patterns in vulnerable individuals. For those without such history, starting with a modest 12:12 (12 hours fasting, 12 hours eating) pattern and gradually extending the fasting window allows your body to adapt gracefully.

Key Takeaways

- The quarter-quarter-half plate method, half vegetables, quarter protein, quarter complex carbohydrates, provides a simple framework for stable blood sugar eating.
- Consistent meal timing (breakfast, regular meals, time-restricted eating window) aligns eating patterns with your circadian rhythm, optimising insulin sensitivity.
- Specific foods, oily fish, leafy greens, legumes, fermented foods, and eggs, simultaneously stabilise blood sugar and provide nutrients essential for mood regulation.
- Intermittent fasting activates autophagy and AMPK/sirtuin pathways, increasing BDNF and enhancing cognitive resilience while improving insulin sensitivity.
- Avoiding common pitfalls (isolated carbohydrates, late-night eating, processed "healthy" foods) prevents metabolic destabilisation and mood swings.

Next Steps

You now have the foundational eating strategies for blood sugar stability. But eating patterns exist within a broader dietary context, the types of fats you consume, the degree to which you process your food, and the environmental exposures you encounter all influence your metabolic health. This shift has serious consequences for inflammation, insulin resistance, and mental health. Understanding the impact of seed oils, and how to make simple substitutions, represents another powerful lever for optimising your metabolism and protecting your brain.

References

Evert, A. B., Dennison, M., Gardner, C. D., Garvey, W. T., Lau, K. H. K., MacLeod, J., … & Yancy, W. S. (2019). Nutrition therapy for adults with diabetes or prediabetes: A consensus report. *Diabetes Care*, 42(5), 731–754. https://doi.org/10.2337/dci19-0014

Lowe, C. J., Reichelt, A. C., & Hall, P. A. (2019). The prefrontal cortex and obesity: A health neuroscience perspective. *Trends in Cognitive Sciences*, 23(4), 349–361. https://doi.org/10.1016/j.tics.2019.01.005

Wilkinson, M. J., Manoogian, E. N., Zadourian, A., Lo, H., Fakhouri, S., Shoghi, A., … & Taub, P. R. (2020). Ten-hour time-restricted eating reduces weight, blood pressure, and atherogenic lipids in patients with metabolic syndrome. *Cell Metabolism*, 31(1), 92–104. https://doi.org/10.1016/j.cmet.2019.11.004

Anton, S. D., Moehl, K., Donahoo, W. T., Marosi, K., Lee, S. A., Mainous, A. G., … & Mattson, M. P. (2018). Flipping the metabolic switch: Understanding and applying the health benefits of fasting. *Obesity*, 26(2), 254–268. https://doi.org/10.1002/oby.22090

Mattson, M. P., Arumugam, T. V., & Guo, Z. (2018). Hallmarks of brain aging: Adaptive and pathological modification by metabolic states. *Cell Metabolism*, 27(6), 1176–1199. https://doi.org/10.1016/j.cmet.2018.05.012

Moro, T., Tinsley, G., Bianco, A., Marcolin, G., Pacelli, Q. F., Battaglia, G., … & Paoli, A. (2016). Effects of eight weeks of time-restricted feeding (16/8) on basal metabolism, maximal strength, body composition, inflammation, and cardiovascular risk factors in resistance-trained males. *Journal of Translational Medicine*, 14(1), 290. https://doi.org/10.1186/s12967-016-1044-2

Chapter 9: Seed Oils, Inflammation, and Blood Sugar

The Fat Revolution You Never Chose

Introduction: A Dramatic Dietary Shift

Blood sugar is often discussed as though it exists in isolation, but your metabolic health depends on the quality of the fats you consume just as much as the carbohydrates you eat. Over the past century, dietary fat consumption has shifted dramatically in Western countries. Traditional animal fats and tropical oils, lard, butter, tallow, coconut oil, have been largely displaced by industrially produced seed oils: soybean oil, canola oil, sunflower oil, corn oil, and cottonseed oil. These oils are inexpensive to produce, have a long shelf life, and were once believed to be healthier than saturated fats. More recent research has complicated this picture. Understanding the impact of seed oils on inflammation, insulin resistance, and mental health is essential for anyone seeking to stabilise their mood and protect their brain.

The Omega-6 to Omega-3 Imbalance

The primary concern with seed oils relates to their extremely high content of omega-6 polyunsaturated fatty acids (PUFAs), particularly linoleic acid. Omega-6 fats are not inherently unhealthy, your body requires them in small amounts. The problem is one of proportion and processing. Human physiology evolved with a dietary ratio of omega-6 to omega-3 fatty acids of approximately 1:1 to 4:1. Your body developed mechanisms to handle this balance, with omega-6 and omega-3 fats competing for the same metabolic pathways.

In today's Western diet, this ratio has ballooned to between 15:1 and 20:1, driven almost entirely by massive increases in seed oil consumption. This imbalance matters deeply. Omega-6 promotes the production of pro-inflammatory eicosanoids, while omega-3 fats produce anti-inflammatory compounds. A chronically pro-inflammatory state is associated with insulin resistance, mood disorders, cognitive decline, and many chronic diseases. Your body is essentially drowning in inflammatory signals while lacking the anti-inflammatory compounds needed to restore balance.

Seed Oil Inflammation and the Brain

Inflammation is now recognised as a central mechanism in depression, anxiety, and other mood disorders. Elevated inflammatory markers, including interleukin-6 (IL-6), tumour necrosis factor-alpha (TNF-α), and C-reactive protein (CRP), are consistently found in individuals with depression, and reducing inflammation through dietary and lifestyle interventions has been shown to improve mood in multiple clinical trials.

High seed oil consumption drives inflammation through several mechanisms. First, the polyunsaturated fats in seed oils are chemically unstable, oxidising during storage and cooking. Second, once ingested, these oxidised fats incorporate into your cell membranes, including the membranes of your brain cells, creating a pro-inflammatory cellular environment. Third, these oxidised fats disrupt immune signalling cascades, activating your immune system in ways that your body perceives as threatening. The brain, with its exceptionally high fat content, is particularly vulnerable to the effects of pro-inflammatory fatty acid imbalances.

A Critical Distinction: Thermal Oxidation

The 2026 scientific consensus on seed oils requires an important distinction between unheated consumption and thermal degradation. Major health bodies, including the 2026 Dietary Guidelines for Americans, maintain that unheated seed oils do not inherently cause systemic inflammation. However, the critical caveat involves **thermal oxidation**.

Seed oils contain multiple double bonds in their chemical structure (high polyunsaturation), making them highly unstable at the high temperatures involved in deep-frying, commercial baking, and industrial food processing. Thermal stress triggers lipid peroxidation, generating reactive and highly toxic aldehydes, most notably **4-hydroxynonenal (4-HNE)** and various peroxide radicals. These thermally generated compounds are highly bioavailable; upon ingestion they cross the blood-brain barrier, activate NF-κB inflammatory signalling, cause endothelial dysfunction, and promote neuroinflammation. The psychiatric risk associated with seed oils is therefore primarily dictated by industrial processing and high-heat cooking rather than the raw, unoxidised oil itself.

Virgin Olive Oil: A Neuroprotective Contrast

In sharp contrast to refined seed oils, **virgin olive oil (VOO)** exhibits deep neuroprotective properties. A 2026 prospective cohort study from the PREDIMED-Plus trial, tracking over 650 older adults at high risk for cognitive decline over two years, found that high VOO consumption was strongly associated with preserved and improved cognitive function, mediated through greater gut microbial diversity. Crucially, increased consumption of refined common olive oil (COO), which is stripped of phenolic compounds during industrial refining, correlated with reduced microbial diversity and accelerated cognitive decline.

The difference is chemical. VOO is rich in phenolic compounds, specifically **hydroxytyrosol**, **oleuropein**, and **tyrosol**, which are stripped away during the refining processes used to produce COO and industrial seed oils. These polyphenols readily cross the blood-brain barrier to directly inhibit beta-amyloid plaque aggregation, prevent tau fibrillisation, reduce oxidative stress, and downregulate pro-inflammatory cytokines. Most importantly, a gut-brain mediation pathway was identified: VOO consumption elevated the gut taxon *Adlercreutzia*, a beneficial microorganism that served as a direct biological mediator bridging VOO consumption to positive cognitive outcomes. This finding demonstrates that VOO's neuroprotection operates not merely through direct antioxidant mechanisms, but through a bidirectional brain-gut microbiota axis, your microbiome becomes healthier, and your mood and cognition improve as a direct consequence.

A Dietary Fats Comparison

Different fats have dramatically different effects on your metabolic and neurological health. Understanding these differences allows you to make strategic substitutions:

Virgin Olive Oil (VOO): High monounsaturated fatty acid (oleic acid) content and rich phenolic compounds make it extremely stable and neuroprotective. It preserves cognition, supports microbiome diversity, and reduces neuroinflammation.

Thermally Oxidised Seed Oils: High polyunsaturated content makes them highly unstable at cooking temperatures. They generate 4-HNE and lipid peroxides that activate inflammatory signalling and cause neuroinflammation.

Unheated Seed Oils: When not heated, they remain intact and are neutral to moderately beneficial, potentially lowering LDL cholesterol without the inflammatory effects of oxidised versions.

Refined Common Olive Oil (COO): Although more stable than seed oils, refining strips away phenolic compounds, reducing neuroprotective benefits and potentially contributing to reduced microbial diversity.

Practical Guidance on Fats

Rather than attempting to eliminate all seed oils overnight (which is unrealistic in modern life), a practical approach focuses on strategic substitutions:

Cook with stable fats. Olive oil (extra virgin, for low-to-medium heat), coconut oil, butter, and ghee are more stable at cooking temperatures and do not produce the same oxidative by-products as seed oils. This single change, switching cooking oils, eliminates one of your largest sources of pro-inflammatory compounds.

Increase omega-3 intake. Regular consumption of oily fish (salmon, sardines, mackerel), flaxseed, chia seeds, and walnuts helps restore a healthier omega-6 to omega-3 balance. This rebalancing reduces systemic inflammation and supports brain health.

Reduce processed food consumption. Seed oils are ubiquitous in packaged foods, fast food, and restaurant cooking. Seed oils dominate the food supply not because they are superior, but because they are inexpensive and have a long shelf life. Reducing overall processed food intake is the most effective single step for reducing seed oil exposure.

Read labels carefully. Seed oils appear under many names including "vegetable oil," "canola oil," "soybean oil," and "sunflower oil." Look for products made with olive oil or coconut oil as alternatives. When eating at restaurants, ask how food is cooked; many establishments now recognise the benefit of cooking with healthier fats and are willing to accommodate requests.

Key Takeaways

- The modern diet's omega-6 to omega-3 ratio (15:1 to 20:1) is drastically elevated due to seed oil consumption, driving systemic inflammation linked to mood disorders and cognitive decline.
- Thermally oxidised seed oils generate 4-HNE and lipid peroxides that cross the blood-brain barrier and activate pro-inflammatory signalling in the brain.
- Virgin olive oil provides neuroprotective phenolic compounds that cross the blood-brain barrier, inhibit amyloid aggregation, and support beneficial gut microbes (Adlercreutzia) that influence mood and cognition.
- Strategic substitutions, cooking with stable fats, increasing omega-3 intake, and reducing processed foods, meaningfully reduce pro-inflammatory seed oil exposure.
- The psychiatric risk associated with seed oils is primarily determined by high-heat processing rather than the unoxidised oil itself.

Next Steps

You have now learned how the foods you choose, from the simple carbohydrates you eat to the fats you cook with, directly influence insulin resistance, systemic inflammation, and mood stability. Yet food represents only part of your metabolic equation. Sleep, how deeply you sleep, how consistently you sleep, and the timing of your sleep, exerts an equally powerful influence on blood sugar regulation and mental health. You will learn how a single night of poor sleep can impair insulin sensitivity as much as days of poor eating, and why protecting your sleep architecture is metabolically non-negotiable for mental health.

References

Simopoulos, A. P. (2016). An increase in the omega-6/omega-3 fatty acid ratio increases the risk for obesity. *Nutrients,* 8(3), 128. https://doi.org/10.3390/nu8030128

Blasbalg, T. L., Hibbeln, J. R., Ramsden, C. E., Majchrzak, S. F., & Rawlings, R. R. (2011). Changes in consumption of omega-3 and omega-6 fatty acids in the United States during the 20th century. *American Journal of Clinical Nutrition*, 93(5), 950–962. https://doi.org/10.3945/ajcn.110.006734

Raison, C. L., Capuron, L., & Miller, A. H. (2006). Cytokines sing the blues: Inflammation and the pathogenesis of depression. *Trends in Immunology*, 27(1), 24–31. https://doi.org/10.1016/j.it.2005.11.006

Barbaresko, J., Koch, M., Schulze, M. B., & Nöthlings, U. (2012). Dietary pattern analysis and type 2 diabetes: A systematic literature review and meta-analysis of observational studies. *The Journal of Nutrition*, 143(3), 336–346. https://doi.org/10.3945/jn.112.169185

Insogna, K. L., Insulander, P., & Keyl, C. (2019). Nutritional determinants of cardiovascular health. *Current Atherosclerosis Reports*, 21(5), 18. https://doi.org/10.1007/s11883-019-0781-y

Vaya, J., & Mahmood, S. (2006). Flavonoid content in leaf extracts of the fig (Ficus carica L.), carob (Ceratonia siliqua L.) and pistachio (Pistacia lentiscus L.) trees. *BioFactors*, 28(1), 17–22. https://doi.org/10.1002/biof.5520280103

U.S. Department of Agriculture and U.S. Department of Health and Human Services. (2026). *Dietary Guidelines for Americans, 2025–2030.*

https://www.realfood.gov

Ni, J., Nishi, S. K., Babio, N., Belzer, C., Vioque, J., Corella, D., … & Salas-Salvadó, J. (2026). Total and different types of olive oil consumption, gut microbiota, and cognitive function changes in older adults. *Microbiome*, 14(1), 68. https://doi.org/10.1186/s40168-025-02306-4

Chapter 10: Sleep's Role in Blood Sugar and Mental Health

The Metabolic Power of Rest

Introduction: Sleep as Metabolic Medicine

Sleep is not a passive state of rest, it is an actively regulated biological process with real effects on metabolism, mood, and cognitive function. If you have read the previous chapters carefully, you understand that blood sugar stability is essential for mental health. But you may not realise that sleep controls blood sugar regulation as powerfully as diet does. The relationship between sleep and blood glucose runs in both directions: poor sleep disrupts blood sugar regulation, and high blood sugar in turn disrupts sleep quality. Optimising sleep is one of the most powerful interventions available for blood sugar and mental health. A single night of poor sleep, defined in research as less than 6 hours, can reduce your insulin sensitivity by 25–30 per cent. This effect is comparable to eating a high-sugar diet for several days. This means that even in people who eat impeccably, chronic sleep deprivation can drive blood sugar instability, insulin resistance, and the mood disturbances that follow.

How Sleep Disruption Destabilises Your Blood Sugar

Sleep exerts its metabolic effects through multiple hormonal pathways. Understanding these pathways illuminates why sleep is non-negotiable for mental health:

Cortisol rhythm. During healthy sleep, cortisol follows a predictable rhythm, low at night, rising gradually in the early morning to initiate waking and provide energy for the day. Sleep deprivation disrupts this rhythm, elevating night-time cortisol and blunting the morning rise. Elevated cortisol at night stimulates glucose release from your liver, raising blood sugar during a period when it should be low. This nocturnal blood sugar elevation fragments your sleep further, creating a vicious cycle of poor sleep and metabolic chaos.

Growth hormone. Deep (slow-wave) sleep triggers the release of growth hormone, which promotes tissue repair, supports insulin sensitivity, and helps regulate blood sugar. Chronic sleep deprivation suppresses growth hormone release, impairing your body's capacity to metabolise glucose and maintain insulin sensitivity. Without adequate deep sleep, your metabolism enters a catabolic state, tissue repair stalls, and metabolic resilience declines.

Ghrelin and leptin. Sleep deprivation elevates ghrelin (the hunger hormone) and suppresses leptin (the satiety hormone), creating powerful biological cravings for high-sugar, high-carbohydrate foods. This is one reason why tired individuals consistently make poorer dietary choices, the neurochemistry of sleep deprivation drives sugar cravings. Your fatigued brain is literally signalling that it needs quick energy (glucose), leading to a cascade of poor decisions that worsen metabolic dysfunction.

Sleep and Emotional Regulation

The links between sleep and mental health are extensive and well-established. Insomnia is both a symptom and a risk factor for depression and anxiety. Poor sleep impairs emotional regulation by disrupting prefrontal cortical function, the brain region responsible for rational thinking and emotional control, while simultaneously amplifying amygdala reactivity, your brain's fear and threat-detection centre. This produces a state of heightened emotional reactivity, reduced stress tolerance, and impaired decision-making. Notably, these symptoms are identical to those produced by blood sugar instability, suggesting that sleep deprivation damages mental health through metabolic pathways.

The Growth Hormone Gateway: A New Mechanistic Understanding

A landmark 2025 study published in *Cell* by researchers at UC Berkeley has provided the most precise molecular explanation yet for why sleep architecture is so central to metabolic and mental health. Growth hormone (GH), essential for muscle repair, lipid metabolism, bone density, and insulin sensitivity, is released almost exclusively during the deepest phases of non-REM (slow-wave) sleep. The study mapped a precise neurological feedback loop in your hypothalamus that governs this process.

During deep sleep, your brain actively suppresses **somatostatin** (which inhibits GH release) while simultaneously upregulating **Growth Hormone-Releasing Hormone (GHRH)**, allowing large, restorative pulses of GH to enter circulation. Crucially, as GH accumulates, it directly stimulates the **locus coeruleus**, the brainstem region responsible for alertness, noradrenergic tone, and autonomic stress responses. This mechanism explains the bidirectional link between sleep quality and next-day cognition and mood: high-quality deep sleep produces maximum GH release, which activates the locus coeruleus, resulting in optimal cognitive focus, emotional regulation, and glucose tolerance the following day.

The reverse cascade is equally powerful. If deep sleep is truncated by stress, alcohol, environmental light, or blood sugar crashes during the night, somatostatin suppression fails, GH release is severely blunted, tissue repair stalls, and systemic insulin resistance skyrockets the following day. An epidemiological study of over 318,000 US adults found that sleeping 5 hours or less was strongly associated with higher rates of diagnosed depression. This mechanism, confirmed across multiple studies, establishes protecting slow-wave sleep architecture as a metabolic imperative, not merely a lifestyle preference.

Practical Strategies for Better Sleep

You cannot control whether your brain releases growth hormone, but you can create the conditions that allow it to do so:

Maintain a consistent sleep schedule. Going to bed and waking at the same time every day, including weekends, anchors your circadian rhythm and improves both sleep quality and metabolic health. Your body thrives on predictability; consistency is far more powerful than sleeping in on weekends.

Create a dark, cool sleep environment. Light suppresses melatonin production, the hormone that initiates sleep. Keep your bedroom as dark as possible (blackout curtains, eye mask) and maintain a temperature of approximately 18–20°C (65–68°F) for optimal sleep quality. A cooler room facilitates the slight drop in core body temperature necessary for deep sleep initiation.

Avoid screens for at least one hour before bed. Blue light from phones, tablets, and televisions suppresses melatonin and delays sleep onset. Use blue-light-blocking glasses if you must use screens in the evening, or switch to warm lighting that mimics the red-orange wavelengths of sunset.

Avoid large meals and alcohol within three hours of bedtime. Both interfere with sleep architecture. Alcohol may make you drowsy initially, but it fragments sleep in the second half of the night, preventing deep sleep and disrupting your cortisol rhythm. Large meals force your digestive system to work during sleep, raising core body temperature.

Address blood sugar before bed. A small protein-and-fat-rich snack before bed, such as a few nuts, a small amount of cheese, or a spoonful of almond butter, can prevent hypoglycaemic episodes during the night that fragment sleep and elevate nocturnal cortisol. The goal is stable glucose throughout the night, not complete fasting.

Chrononutrition: When You Eat Matters as Much as What You Eat

While most nutritional science focuses on *what* you eat, macronutrient ratios, micronutrient content, food quality, an emerging field called **chrononutrition** reveals that *when* you eat deeply affects both metabolic health and mood. Your body is not simply a collection of biochemical reactions happening in isolation. Rather, your physiology operates on multiple interlocking circadian rhythms, roughly 24-hour biological cycles that regulate insulin secretion, cortisol release, hormonal cycles, and the synthesis of mood-regulating neurotransmitters.

Your body's master clock is located in the **suprachiasmatic nucleus (SCN)** of your hypothalamus. This clock is synchronised by external time signals called **zeitgebers** (literally, "time-givers"). Sunlight exposure is the primary zeitgeber, but **meal timing is a secondary but powerful circadian signal** that influences peripheral clocks in your metabolic tissues, the liver, pancreas, adipose tissue, and even the brain itself.

When food is consumed outside normal waking hours, particularly late evening or night, your body's internal rhythm becomes desynchronised. Your pancreas, liver, and adipose tissue are signalled to perform metabolic work (digestion, insulin secretion, nutrient storage) at a time when their circadian programmes expect them to be in a fasted, quiescent state. This chronobiological mismatch impairs insulin sensitivity dramatically: the same food consumed late in the evening produces a 25–40 per cent greater blood sugar response than when consumed in the morning.

Time-Restricted Eating (TRE) aligns your eating with your brain's natural circadian patterns. By confining food intake to a specific 8–10 hour window during waking hours, you synchronise your peripheral metabolic clocks, improve insulin sensitivity, enhance post-prandial glucose clearance, and stabilise hormonal rhythms. Studies demonstrate that individuals practising TRE show improved fasting glucose, reduced HbA1c, and decreased cardiovascular disease markers even without weight loss.

Chronotype Variation and Meal Timing Alignment

A particularly important discovery involves **chronotype variation**, your individual biological tendency to be an early-riser ("early chronotype") or evening-preference eater ("late chronotype"). Continuous glucose monitoring reveals that individuals with a late chronotype exhibit higher and more erratic glucose variability compared to early eaters consuming identical meals. Eating in misalignment with your chronotype creates metabolic chaos; your pancreatic and hepatic clocks are essentially out of sync with your meal timing. This chronotype-meal misalignment creates particularly severe psychiatric consequences. Precision Time-Restricted Eating (TRE) protocols are now being integrated into psychiatric care frameworks, with protocols targeting individuals' specific chronotype to restrict food intake to their optimal circadian windows. This practice stabilises peripheral metabolic clocks, reduces glycaemic volatility, and decreases autonomic arousal, specifically alleviating symptoms of atypical depression, anxiety, and insomnia.

The **cortisol awakening response (CAR)**, the normal rise in cortisol immediately after waking, is enhanced by eating breakfast early and blunted by fasting in the morning. Eating breakfast within 30–60 minutes of waking anchors your circadian rhythms and sets a stable metabolic tone for the entire day. Conversely, late-night eating suppresses melatonin synthesis and fragments sleep architecture, creating a vicious cycle where poor sleep worsens insulin sensitivity the following day.

For mental health specifically, circadian misalignment driven by eating late in the day is associated with increased rates of depression and anxiety. Aligning meal timing with your body's natural circadian rhythm, eating most food earlier in the day and finishing eating 2–3 hours before sleep, supports both metabolic resilience and emotional stability.

Key Takeaways

- A single night of poor sleep reduces insulin sensitivity by 25–30 per cent, producing metabolic disruption comparable to days of poor eating.
- Sleep deprivation disrupts cortisol rhythm, suppresses growth hormone, and elevates ghrelin while suppressing leptin, creating a perfect metabolic storm.
- Growth hormone released during deep sleep directly activates the locus coeruleus, optimising next-day cognition, emotional regulation, and glucose tolerance.
- Time-restricted eating synchronises peripheral metabolic clocks, improving insulin sensitivity and stabilising mood even in people who maintain consistent caloric intake.
- Chronotype-aligned meal timing (eating in alignment with whether you are naturally early or late) reduces glucose variability and psychiatric symptoms including depression and anxiety.

Next Steps

You have now explored how diet, fats, and sleep architecture work together to stabilise blood sugar and protect mental health. Yet these lifestyle factors exist within a broader context, the chemical environment surrounding you. Modern life introduces countless synthetic chemicals that your ancestors never encountered. Many of these chemicals directly disrupt the very metabolic and hormonal pathways we have been discussing. You will learn how to assess your chemical load and implement practical strategies to reduce toxic exposure, another powerful lever for protecting your brain and stabilising your mood.

References

Spiegel, K., Tasali, E., Penev, P., & Van Cauter, E. (2004). Brief communication: Sleep curtailment in healthy young men is associated with decreased leptin levels, elevated ghrelin levels, and increased hunger and appetite. *Annals of Internal Medicine*, 141(11), 846–850. https://doi.org/10.7326/0003-4819-141-11-200412070-00008

Leproult, R., & Van Cauter, E. (2010). Role of sleep and sleep loss in hormonal release and metabolism. *Endocrine Development*, 17, 11–21. https://doi.org/10.1159/000262524

Walker, M. P. (2017). *Why we sleep: Unlocking the power of sleep and dreams*. Scribner.

Rao, M. N., Neylan, T. C., Grunfeld, C., Mulligan, K., Schambelan, M., & Schwarz, J. M. (2015). Subchronic sleep restriction causes tissue-specific insulin resistance. *Journal of Clinical Endocrinology & Metabolism*, 100(4), 1664–1671. https://doi.org/10.1210/jc.2014-4053

Sutton, E. F., Beyl, R., Early, K. S., Cefalu, W. T., Ravussin, E., & Peterson, C. M. (2018). Early time-restricted feeding improves insulin sensitivity, blood pressure, and oxidative stress even without weight loss in men with prediabetes. *Cell Metabolism*, 27(6), 1212–1221. https://doi.org/10.1016/j.cmet.2018.04.010

Poggiogalle, E., Jamshed, H., & Peterson, C. M. (2018). Circadian regulation of glucose, lipid, and energy metabolism in humans. *Metabolism: Clinical and Experimental*, 84, 11–27. https://doi.org/10.1016/j.metabol.2017.11.017

Ding, X., & Dan, Y. (2025). Neuroendocrine circuit for sleep-dependent growth hormone release. *Cell*, 188(18), 4968–4979. https://doi.org/10.1016/j.cell.2025.05.039

Chapter 11: Environmental Toxins, Chemicals, and Blood Sugar

The Hidden Metabolic Disruptors Around You

Introduction: The Chemical World We Inherit

The effort you put into diet and sleep exists within a chemical context your grandparents never encountered. Since the mid-20th century, tens of thousands of synthetic compounds have entered the environment through food packaging, pesticides, cleaning products, personal care items, and water supplies. Many interact with your hormonal and metabolic systems in ways that quietly undermine the very changes you are trying to make. This is not cause for despair, it is cause for practical, targeted action.

A specific class of chemicals, **endocrine-disrupting chemicals (EDCs)**, has attracted particular scientific attention for their ability to interfere with hormone signalling, including the insulin and cortisol pathways that regulate blood sugar. Exposures that once seemed trivially small have been shown, through decades of research, to have measurable effects on metabolic function, mood, and neurological health. Understanding these threats and implementing practical strategies to reduce exposure represents another essential layer of metabolic protection.

Key Endocrine-Disrupting Chemicals

Bisphenol A (BPA) and its substitutes. Found in some plastics, food can linings, and thermal paper receipts, BPA mimics oestrogen and has been shown to impair pancreatic beta-cell function, reduce insulin sensitivity, and contribute to obesity. BPA has been linked to anxiety-like behaviour and mood changes in animal studies. The catch is that BPA-free alternatives often contain bisphenol S (BPS) or bisphenol F (BPF), which appear to have similar endocrine-disrupting properties. The industry simply replaced one problematic chemical with another chemically similar alternative.

Phthalates. Used in plastics, personal care products, and food packaging, phthalates interfere with testosterone and thyroid hormone function. They have been associated with insulin resistance and increased abdominal fat, the type of visceral adiposity most associated with metabolic dysfunction. Phthalates are particularly concerning because they leach into food and personal care products, creating continuous low-level exposure.

Pesticides and herbicides. Organophosphate pesticides, used extensively in conventional agriculture, have been linked to impaired glucose metabolism and increased risk of type 2 diabetes. Glyphosate, the world's most widely used herbicide, is an emerging area of concern, with research suggesting effects on gut microbiome diversity and inflammatory pathways. Your gut microbiome, as discussed in previous chapters, directly influences mood and metabolic health.

Heavy metals. Lead, mercury, cadmium, and arsenic are present in contaminated water, certain fish species, industrial emissions, and old paint. These metals interfere with insulin signalling, impair mitochondrial function, and contribute to neurological damage that affects mood and cognitive function. Heavy metal exposure during childhood has been particularly associated with neurodevelopmental effects.

Practical Strategies to Reduce Your Toxic Load

While complete avoidance of all environmental toxins is currently impossible, you can reduce your exposure through strategic choices:

Eat organic when possible. Prioritise organic versions of produce with the highest pesticide residues, the "dirty dozen," including strawberries, spinach, apples, and grapes. These fruits and vegetables, when conventionally grown, receive frequent pesticide applications and retain more residues. Organic produce, by contrast, is grown without synthetic pesticides, reducing your exposure substantially.

Filter drinking water. A high-quality carbon or reverse-osmosis filter removes chlorine, fluoride, heavy metals, and many pharmaceutical residues from tap water. Your water source is a direct route of chemical exposure; filtering this removes a major source of toxic exposure.

Avoid plastics in contact with food. Store food in glass, stainless steel, or ceramic containers. Never heat food in plastic containers, as heat dramatically increases chemical leaching from plastics into your food. Microwave heating is particularly problematic; the combination of heat and microwave radiation accelerates BPA and phthalate leaching.

Choose natural personal care products. Look for products free of phthalates, parabens, and synthetic fragrances. Your skin is highly permeable; chemicals applied topically are readily absorbed. Personal care products represent a direct route of chemical exposure that you control completely.

Increase fibre and antioxidants. Many toxins bind to fibre in your gut and are excreted rather than absorbed. Antioxidants support your liver's detoxification pathways, enhancing your body's capacity to eliminate toxins. Cruciferous vegetables (broccoli, Brussels sprouts, cabbage) are particularly effective at supporting liver detoxification.

Microplastics and PFAS: The New Environmental Threats

Among the most recent and concerning environmental toxins with direct implications for metabolic psychiatry are **microplastics** and **per- and polyfluoroalkyl substances (PFAS)**. Both are ubiquitous in the modern environment, accumulate in human tissues including the brain, and actively disrupt glucose metabolism and insulin signalling.

Microplastics are plastic particles smaller than 5 millimetres that originate from the breakdown of larger plastic products and from the intentional use of microbeads in cosmetics and personal care products. Adults now ingest approximately 250 grams of microplastics annually, a startling figure that illustrates how completely plastic has infiltrated the food supply. A 2025 study published in *Nature Medicine* documented that nanoplastics cross the blood-brain barrier and accumulate in neural tissue at concentrations 7–30 times higher than in liver or kidney, with even greater accumulation found in brain samples from individuals with dementia. Once in your brain, they trigger neuroinflammation through microglial activation, generate reactive oxygen species (ROS), and impair mitochondrial function.

Most alarmingly, microplastic exposure causes **epigenetic silencing of essential antioxidant genes**, specifically SOD1 (superoxide dismutase 1) and CAT (catalase), the critical enzymes protecting your neurons from free radical damage. This epigenetic repression exhausts your brain's defensive capacity against oxidative stress. Exposure to microplastics in animal models also impairs insulin signalling in the brain and reduces the sensitivity of hypothalamic neurons to insulin's satiety signals, promoting dysregulated feeding behaviour and weight gain. The neuroinflammation induced by microplastics mirrors that seen in depression and anxiety disorders, suggesting a direct mechanism linking plastic exposure to mood dysfunction.

PFAS ("forever chemicals") are synthetic compounds used in non-stick coatings, food packaging, stain-resistant fabrics, and firefighting foams. A 2026 systematic review confirmed that PFAS exposure aggressively disrupts beta-cell function and insulin secretion alongside glucose homeostasis. Unlike most organic pollutants, PFAS are not broken down in your body and accumulate indefinitely in your liver, kidneys, and serum, and have been detected in human brain samples. PFAS directly impair insulin secretion and insulin signalling in peripheral tissues and, critically, disrupt thyroid hormone metabolism. The combined insult reduces expression of essential glucose transporters (GLUT3 and GLUT4), creating profound neuronal energy deficit directly linked to mood instability and cognitive decline. Since thyroid hormones regulate metabolic rate and are essential for mood stability, PFAS-induced thyroid dysfunction contributes to both metabolic dysfunction and psychiatric symptoms.

Animal and clinical evidence suggests that both microplastics and PFAS impair glucose tolerance, increase insulin resistance, promote systemic inflammation, and contribute to the metabolic dysfunction underlying depression and anxiety. Exposure occurs through drinking water (particularly from non-stick cookware and food packaging), inhalation of air-borne microplastics, and consumption of contaminated foods.

Reducing Microplastic and PFAS Exposure

While complete avoidance is currently impossible, reducing exposure is possible:

- Filter drinking water with a high-quality filter capable of removing PFAS compounds.
- Avoid non-stick cookware; stainless steel and cast iron are preferable and do not leach PFAS.
- Choose organic foods when possible; organically grown foods have lower pesticide and PFAS residues.
- Reduce dependence on packaged convenience foods; home-cooked meals eliminate much of the microplastic and PFAS exposure from food packaging and processing.
- Avoid single-use plastics; choose glass, stainless steel, and ceramic when possible.

Key Takeaways

- Endocrine-disrupting chemicals (BPA, phthalates, pesticides, heavy metals) directly impair pancreatic beta-cell function, disrupt insulin signalling, and promote systemic inflammation.
- Microplastics accumulate in brain tissue, trigger neuroinflammation, silence antioxidant genes, and impair insulin signalling in neurons, directly contributing to mood dysfunction.
- PFAS ("forever chemicals") permanently accumulate in tissues, disrupt thyroid hormone metabolism, and impair insulin secretion, creating neuronal energy deficits linked to depression and anxiety.
- Strategic reductions in chemical exposure (organic foods, water filtration, avoiding plastics, natural personal care) significantly decrease toxic burden without requiring complete life changes.
- Chemical exposure represents a modifiable risk factor; reducing exposure enhances metabolic health and mental resilience.

Next Steps

You have now explored several major dietary and environmental factors influencing blood sugar regulation and mental health: the foods you eat, the fats you consume, your sleep patterns, and the chemical exposures you incur. Yet there is one more environmental factor now widely recognised as affecting metabolic and neurological health: the electromagnetic fields (EMFs) surrounding you. In the next chapter, we examine the evidence regarding EMF exposure, its effects on insulin signalling and sleep, and practical precautionary strategies for reducing exposure. While the science here is still evolving, understanding these mechanisms and implementing simple protective measures represents another low-cost, zero-risk intervention for optimising your metabolic and mental health.

References

Trasande, L., Attina, T. M., & Blustein, J. (2012). Association between urinary bisphenol A concentration and obesity prevalence in children and adolescents. *JAMA*, 308(11), 1113–1121. https://doi.org/10.1001/jama.2012.8827

Mnif, W., Hassine, A. I. H., Bouaziz, A., Bartegi, A., Thomas, O., & Roig, B. (2011). Effect of endocrine disruptor pesticides: A review. *International Journal of Environmental Research and Public Health*, 8(6), 2265–2303. https://doi.org/10.3390/ijerph8062265

Trasande, L., Zoeller, R. T., Hass, U., Kortenkamp, A., Grandjean, P., Myers, J. P., … & Heindel, J. J. (2015). Estimating burden and disease costs of exposure to endocrine-disrupting chemicals in the European Union. *Journal of Clinical Endocrinology & Metabolism,* 100(4), 1245–1255. https://doi.org/10.1210/jc.2014-3957

Ragusa, A., Svelato, A., Santacroce, C., Catalano, P., Notarstefano, V., Carnevali, O., … & Giorgini, A. (2021). Plasticenta: First evidence of microplastics in human placenta. *Environment International*, 146, 106274. https://doi.org/10.1016/j.envint.2020.106274

Jönsson, B. A. G., Salihovic, S., Kärrman, A., Lind, P. M., Lindh, C. H., Jakobsson, K., Valeri, L., Andersson, E. M., Åsling, A., & Lind, L. (2023).

Associations between per- and polyfluoroalkyl substances (PFAS) and diabetes in two population-based cohort studies from Sweden. *Journal of Exposure Science & Environmental Epidemiology,* 33, 748–759. https://doi.org/10.1038/s41370-023-00566-6

Wang, Z., DeWitt, J. C., Higgins, C. P., & Cousins, I. T. (2017). A never-ending story of per- and polyfluoroalkyl substances (PFASs)? *Environmental Science & Technology,* 51(5), 2508–2518. https://doi.org/10.1021/acs.est.6b04806

Nihart, A. J., Garcia, M. A., El Hayek, E., Liu, R., Olewine, M., & Campen, M. J. (2025). Bioaccumulation of microplastics in decedent human brains. *Nature Medicine*, 31(4), 1114–1119. https://doi.org/10.1038/s41591-024-03453-1

India Aldana, S., Valvi, D., & Yu, X. (2026). Associations of perfluoroalkyl and polyfluoroalkyl substances with markers of glycaemic control, insulin secretion and sensitivity, and diabetes risk: A systematic review and meta-analyses. *eClinicalMedicine.* https://doi.org/10.1016/j.eclinm.2025.103747

Chapter 12: Electromagnetic Fields, Blood Sugar, and Mood

The Invisible Environment and Your Brain

Introduction: An Unseen Metabolic Factor

Electromagnetic fields (EMFs) are invisible areas of energy, often referred to as radiation, that are associated with the use of electrical power and various natural and man-made light sources. They exist on a spectrum of frequencies, from extremely low frequency (ELF) fields generated by power lines and household appliances, to radiofrequency (RF) fields emitted by mobile phones, Wi-Fi routers, and 5G networks. Non-ionising radiation, which includes RF-EMFs from wireless devices, is now a constant and unavoidable feature of modern life. The electromagnetic environment today is thousands of times more saturated than it was just three decades ago. For someone seeking to optimise blood sugar and mental health, understanding the biological mechanisms by which EMF exposure affects metabolism and learning to adopt a precautionary approach to exposure represents another evidence-informed lever for brain protection.

Understanding Non-Ionising Radiation and Biological Effects

The distinction between ionising and non-ionising radiation is important. Ionising radiation (from X-rays and nuclear sources) has enough energy to knock electrons from atoms, directly damaging DNA. Non-ionising radiation cannot do this directly. However, the evidence suggests it activates cellular stress responses through other mechanisms. The mainstream regulatory position holds that non-ionising radiation below established safety thresholds, most commonly the Specific Absorption Rate (SAR) standard, poses no established health risk. Yet a growing body of research, much of it published since 2010 and conducted in Central and Eastern European research institutions, suggests that chronic EMF exposure may have subtle biological effects that current safety standards, which are based largely on thermal effects (heating), do not adequately account for. This divergence between regulatory reassurance and emerging mechanism-based science reflects a genuine scientific uncertainty, not scientific consensus.

Oxidative Stress and Insulin Receptor Impairment

One of the most thoroughly researched mechanisms linking EMF exposure to metabolic dysfunction is the induction of **oxidative stress**, an imbalance between free radical production and your body's antioxidant capacity. Several studies suggest that EMF exposure, particularly radiofrequency EMFs, activates **voltage-gated calcium channels** in cell membranes. When these channels open, excess calcium floods into cells, triggering a cascade of metabolic events: mitochondrial stress, activation of enzymes that generate reactive oxygen species (ROS), and ultimately oxidative damage to cell structures.

This oxidative stress has particular relevance to blood sugar regulation. Your insulin receptor is a protein embedded in cell membranes, and its function depends on precise redox balance. When your cells are exposed to elevated ROS, your insulin receptor's signalling machinery becomes impaired, a process called **insulin receptor oxidation**. The result is reduced insulin sensitivity: even if your blood insulin levels are elevated, your cells respond less effectively to that signal, leading to chronically higher blood glucose. Additionally, oxidative stress in your pancreatic beta cells impairs their function, reducing insulin secretion capacity. This dual effect, worsening both insulin secretion and insulin sensitivity, makes EMF-induced oxidative stress a plausible link between chronic wireless device exposure and metabolic dysfunction.

Blue Light, Melatonin, and Sleep-Glucose Disruption

EMF exposure, particularly from screens emitting **blue light**, suppresses melatonin production in your pineal gland. This effect has been well-documented in chronobiology research: the blue wavelengths (approximately 460–480 nm) emitted by smartphone screens, computer monitors, and LED lighting suppress melatonin via melanopsin receptors in your retina, effectively communicating to your body that it is still daytime. The consequence cascades through multiple systems.

Melatonin, as discussed in Chapter 10, is far more than a sleep hormone: it is a potent antioxidant and mitochondrial protector. When melatonin production is suppressed by evening screen exposure, several things happen simultaneously. First, your sleep becomes fragmented and shallow, melatonin is essential for sleep architecture, particularly for maintaining slow-wave (deep) sleep. Second, without melatonin's protection, mitochondrial oxidative stress increases through the night. Third, sleep fragmentation triggers nocturnal cortisol elevation, disrupting the normal cortisol dip that allows your liver's glucose production to be suppressed. The result is waking with elevated fasting blood glucose and a disrupted cortisol rhythm.

This is why the practical step of removing screens from your bedroom and stopping all screen use 60–90 minutes before sleep has such disproportionate impact on both sleep quality and fasting blood glucose. The magnitude of effect often surprises people: sleep onset latency (time to fall asleep) frequently improves within days, and morning fasting glucose often drops 10–20 mg/dL within a week of consistent screen avoidance before bed. This simple change, establishing a technology-free transition period before sleep, may be among the highest-leverage interventions available for sleep quality and metabolic health.

Night-Time Device Use: Exposure During Your Most Vulnerable Period

The habit of sleeping with a mobile phone beside your bed, powered on, with Wi-Fi enabled, represents a particularly intensive EMF exposure during the period of greatest metabolic vulnerability: sleep. During sleep, your body's ability to manage oxidative stress is somewhat impaired, and the regulatory systems that maintain glucose homeostasis are in a different state than during wakefulness. Your sympathetic nervous system is less active, and parasympathetic tone (rest-and-digest) is elevated. This is the state in which your body most needs protection from inflammatory and oxidative stress.

Night-time EMF exposure from a bedside phone contributes to this stress in three ways: through direct oxidative stress activation (voltage-gated calcium channel effects), through melatonin suppression if the phone's indicator light or any notifications trigger sleep arousals, and through activation of your stress response if EMF exposure activates your body's threat-detection systems. The cumulative effect is a night of lower-quality sleep, higher nocturnal cortisol, and a morning waking state characterised by elevated fasting glucose, impaired mental clarity, and reduced stress resilience. This outcome directly undermines the metabolic improvements you are seeking through diet and sleep optimisation.

Circadian Rhythm Disruption and Metabolic Dysregulation

Beyond the direct effects on melatonin and sleep architecture, chronic EMF exposure, particularly the irregular, pulsed nature of wireless signals from mobile networks, appears to disrupt your body's **circadian timing system**. Your circadian rhythm is the master regulator of hundreds of physiological processes, including the glucose-regulation cascade discussed throughout this book. When circadian rhythm is disrupted, multiple metabolic clocks become uncoordinated.

The practical manifestation is often subtle: slightly elevated fasting blood glucose, reduced afternoon energy despite adequate sleep duration, and mood instability that doesn't seem to have an obvious external cause. These are signs of circadian phase disruption. Your body's internal clocks gradually desynchronise when exposed to environmental signals that contradict the light-dark cycle, and constant low-level EMF exposure may be one such signal. By protecting your circadian alignment, you maintain the metabolic synchronisation essential for stable mood and cognitive function.

Precautionary Strategies for EMF Reduction

The scientific consensus on EMF health effects continues to evolve. Given the evidence for oxidative stress mechanisms, melatonin suppression, and circadian disruption, and given that EMF reduction carries no downside, the most practical and cautious approach is to implement the following strategies:

Create device-free bedrooms. Keep mobile phones, tablets, and wireless devices out of your bedroom, or place them in aeroplane mode. This eliminates the most sensitive period of exposure, sleep, when your body is least able to defend against oxidative stress. If you rely on your phone as an alarm, use a traditional alarm clock instead. The improvement in sleep quality and fasting blood glucose often justifies this change alone, within days of implementation.

Use wired internet connections where practical. For devices that are stationary (computers, smart televisions), use Ethernet cables instead of Wi-Fi. Wi-Fi exposure is continuous and whole-body; wired connections eliminate this exposure for devices that don't need mobility. For households with young children, this change is particularly important, as smaller bodies absorb proportionally more RF energy than adult bodies.

Adopt aeroplane mode protocols. Use aeroplane mode on your mobile phone during focused work, meals, and the evening hours. Aeroplane mode disables all wireless transmission, reducing both radiation exposure and the constant low-level activation of your nervous system that wireless signals appear to trigger. The practical benefit is often improved focus during work and better sleep preparation in the evening.

Establish a screen curfew before sleep. Establish a screen-free period starting 60–90 minutes before bed. This protects melatonin production, reduces blue light exposure, and allows your nervous system to settle into parasympathetic tone. The combined effect on sleep quality and next-morning fasting glucose is often profound. Within a week, most people notice improved sleep quality and stable morning energy.

Limit cumulative device exposure. Rather than viewing EMF reduction as all-or-nothing, recognise that dose matters: 30 minutes of screen time held to your ear is more problematic than 8 hours of laptop use at arm's distance. Use speakerphone or wired headsets when possible; keep phones away from your body when not in active use. During working hours, regular breaks from screens allow both visual strain and EMF exposure to decrease.

Assess your residential EMF environment. High-density wireless exposure varies considerably depending on your living situation. Flats in apartment buildings with multiple neighbours' Wi-Fi networks will have greater ambient

RF exposure than detached homes in rural areas. If you live in a high-EMF environment, device-free bedrooms and EMF reduction at home become more important for protecting your sleep and metabolic health. Some people find modest benefit from EMF-shielding materials for the bedroom, though the evidence for these is less robust than for simple device removal.

Key Takeaways

- Chronic EMF exposure, particularly from wireless devices, may activate oxidative stress pathways that impair insulin receptor signalling and worsen both blood sugar regulation and mood stability.
- Blue light from screens suppresses melatonin production, fragmenting sleep and elevating nocturnal cortisol, a particularly problematic combination for fasting blood glucose control and emotional regulation.
- The most effective practical strategy is to remove wireless devices from your bedroom and establish a screen-free period of 60–90 minutes before sleep, which typically improves sleep quality and reduces morning fasting glucose within days.
- Wired internet connections, aeroplane mode usage, and speakerphone protocols are practical methods to reduce cumulative EMF exposure without sacrificing device functionality.
- For mental health and metabolic optimisation, EMF reduction is a low-cost, zero-risk intervention with emerging mechanism-based evidence and observable practical benefits.

Next Steps

You have now explored a core set of environmental and dietary factors that shape blood sugar regulation and mental health, the foods you choose, the fats you consume, the quality of your sleep, the chemicals surrounding you, and the electromagnetic environment you inhabit. Each exerts a measurable influence on your insulin sensitivity, your glucose levels, and your brain's capacity to regulate mood. But the story does not end here. The chapters ahead examine how sunlight, vitamin D, grounding, nature exposure, physical activity, and the gut-brain axis all converge on the same metabolic pathways, and how optimising each of them creates compounding benefits for both physical and mental wellbeing. Continue to Chapter 13 to explore one of the most under-recognised metabolic interventions available to you: light.

References

Pall, M. L. (2016). Microwave frequency electromagnetic fields (EMFs) produce widespread neuropsychiatric effects including depression. *Journal of Chemical Neuroanatomy*, 75, 43–51. https://doi.org/10.1016/j.jchemneu.2016.01.001

Yakymenko, I., Tsybulin, O., Sidorik, E., Henshel, D., Kyrylenko, O., & Kyrylenko, S. (2016). Oxidative mechanisms of biological activity of low-intensity radiofrequency radiation. *Electromagnetic Biology and Medicine*, 35(2), 186–202. https://doi.org/10.3109/15368378.2015.1043557

Saliev, T., Begimbetova, D., Masoud, A. R., & Matkarimov, B. (2019). Biological effects of non-ionizing electromagnetic fields: Two sides of a coin. *Progress in Biophysics and Molecular Biology*, 141, 25–36. https://doi.org/10.1016/j.pbiomolbio.2018.07.009

Belpomme, D., Campagnac, C., & Irigaray, P. (2015). Reliable disease biomarkers characterizing and identifying electrohypersensitivity and multiple chemical sensitivity as two etiopathogenic aspects of a unique pathological disorder. *Reviews on Environmental Health*, 30(4), 251–271. https://doi.org/10.1515/reveh-2015-0027

Havas, M., Marrongelle, J., Pollner, B., Kelley, E., Rees, C. R. G., & Tully, L. (2010). Provocation study using heart rate variability shows microwave radiation from 2.4 GHz cordless phone affects autonomic nervous system. *European Journal of Oncology Library*, 5, 273–300.

Chang, H. S., Butenhoff, J. L., & Deon, S. D. (2018). Hazard assessment of perfluorooctanesulfonate (PFOS) and its salts. *Reviews of Environmental Contamination and Toxicology*, 243, 1–58. https://doi.org/10.1007/398_2016_10

Chapter 13: Sunlight, Vitamin D, and Blood Sugar Balance

Vitamin D as a Master Metabolic Regulator

Introduction: Understanding Vitamin D's Role

Despite its name, vitamin D is not really a vitamin, it is a prohormone that your body converts into a potent steroid hormone capable of regulating more than 2,000 genes. Deficiency is epidemic: over 40 per cent of Australians are insufficient, and rates are even higher among those with depression or anxiety. Correcting a simple vitamin D deficiency can produce measurable improvements in blood sugar control and mental wellbeing that surprise clinicians accustomed to reaching for a prescription pad first.

The Prohormone That Controls Your Metabolic Destiny

Vitamin D begins its journey through sunlight, not from food. When ultraviolet B (UVB) radiation, specifically wavelengths between 290 and 315 nanometres, strikes your skin, it initiates a biochemical transformation. This light energy converts 7-dehydrocholesterol in your skin into previtamin D3, which then becomes **cholecalciferol** (vitamin D3). Your liver transforms this further into 25-hydroxyvitamin D (calcifediol), the form measured in blood tests and used as the standard marker of your vitamin D status. In your kidneys, a final conversion produces **1,25-dihydroxyvitamin D3** (calcitriol), the most biologically active form. This activated hormone then enters cells throughout your body, binding to the **vitamin D receptor** (VDR), a transcription factor that directly alters which genes are switched on or off, affecting calcium metabolism, immune regulation, cell growth, and metabolic control.

This pathway explains why modern indoor living, routine sunscreen use, reduced midday sunlight, climate-controlled buildings, has created a metabolic vulnerability previous generations never faced.

How Vitamin D Controls Your Pancreas

Vitamin D receptors are abundantly expressed on your pancreatic beta cells, the specialised cells that produce and release insulin. When vitamin D binds to these receptors, it directly influences your insulin gene expression and the cellular machinery responsible for insulin secretion. Research has consistently shown that when vitamin D is deficient, your beta cells respond sluggishly to rising blood glucose: after eating, they secrete less insulin than they should. Additionally, vitamin D influences how well your muscles, fat, and liver cells respond to insulin's signal. When vitamin D is adequate, genes that facilitate glucose uptake become actively expressed. When vitamin D is deficient, this capacity diminishes. The consequence is a dual metabolic impairment: your pancreas fails to secrete adequate insulin, and your cells fail to respond adequately to the insulin that is present. This creates chronically elevated blood glucose, which cascades through your mood, energy, and disease risk as detailed throughout this book.

The Epidemiological Case: Vitamin D and Type 2 Diabetes

Large prospective cohort studies have painted a consistent picture. Individuals in the lowest quartile of vitamin D status, less than 50 nmol/L (20 ng/mL), have a 50–100 per cent increased risk of developing type 2 diabetes compared with those in the highest quartile. Meta-analyses aggregating dozens of studies reveal a dose-response relationship: each 25 nmol/L increase in vitamin D status is associated with approximately a 5–10 per cent reduction in diabetes risk.

Intervention studies strengthen this case. When researchers have given people vitamin D supplementation and followed them prospectively, the results are compelling. Doses of 1,000–4,000 IU daily for 3–6 months consistently improve fasting blood glucose, HbA1c (your 3-month average blood glucose), and HOMA-IR (a calculated measure of insulin resistance). The relationship is particularly pronounced in individuals who are both overweight and vitamin D deficient. Adipose tissue (fat) actively sequesters vitamin D and reduces its availability in your bloodstream, meaning that overweight, vitamin D-deficient individuals often have the most to gain from vitamin D repletion.

Vitamin D and Your Mood: Neuroprotection at the Cellular Level

Your brain is extraordinarily rich in vitamin D receptors. They cluster in the hippocampus (crucial for memory), the prefrontal cortex (essential for emotional regulation and decision-making), and the substantia nigra (where dopamine is produced). Activated vitamin D exerts neuroprotective effects through multiple mechanisms: it reduces neuroinflammation by toning down microglial activation and pro-inflammatory cytokine production, it regulates the synthesis of neurotrophic factors that support neuronal survival and plasticity, and it directly influences the synthesis of serotonin, dopamine, and GABA, your brain's primary mood-regulating neurotransmitters.

The association between low vitamin D and depression is amongst the most robust findings in psychiatry. Multiple meta-analyses have found that individuals with depression have significantly lower vitamin D levels than non-depressed controls, and the association is dose-dependent. Longitudinal studies suggest the relationship is causal: individuals with low baseline vitamin D status develop depression at higher rates over subsequent years. Vitamin D supplementation in deficient individuals with depression has improved mood in several randomised controlled trials, with effect sizes comparable to some standard antidepressant medications.

Seasonal affective disorder (SAD), the depression that characteristically emerges in winter months, particularly at higher latitudes, directly links to reduced sunlight exposure (and thus reduced vitamin D synthesis). The fact that SAD is most prevalent in countries with the lowest winter UVB exposure and shortest daylight hours points to vitamin D's central role. Vitamin D activates the gene encoding **tryptophan hydroxylase 2** (TPH2), the rate-limiting enzyme in serotonin synthesis within the brain. Low vitamin D means lower TPH2 expression, resulting in reduced capacity for serotonin synthesis. Given that serotonin is a master regulator of mood, stress tolerance, and sleep, vitamin D deficiency therefore represents a fundamental constraint on mood stability. Repletion removes this constraint.

Safe Sun Exposure: Practical Guidelines for Your Latitude and Skin

The synthesis of vitamin D through sun exposure depends on your latitude, season, time of day, cloud cover, skin tone, age, and how much skin is exposed. At lower latitudes (closer to the equator), meaningful UVB is available year-round and throughout much of the day. At higher latitudes, meaningful UVB is available only during spring, summer, and early autumn, and only during midday hours (roughly 10 a.m. to 3 p.m.). Cloud cover and air pollution significantly reduce UVB penetration. Darker skin tones require longer exposure times to achieve the same vitamin D synthesis as lighter skin tones because melanin absorbs some of the incident UVB. Your capacity to synthesise vitamin D also declines with age: a 70-year-old requires approximately three to four times longer sun exposure than a 20-year-old to produce the same quantity.

A practical guideline is to aim for 10–30 minutes of direct, midday sunlight on exposed skin (face, arms, and legs) without sunscreen, most days of the week. For someone in Southern Australia in summer, 10–15 minutes suffices. For someone in Scotland in winter, meaningful vitamin D synthesis may not occur even with extended exposure. For someone with darker skin tone, 30–45 minutes may be required year-round.

Importantly, morning and evening walks, whilst not contributing to vitamin D synthesis due to low UVB intensity, are beneficial for a separate reason: they reset your circadian rhythm and increase bright-light exposure, which enhances serotonin synthesis and improves mood. These walks have psychological and circadian benefits independent of vitamin D production, and should be maintained year-round.

Sunscreen, when applied at real-life concentrations, reduces vitamin D synthesis by approximately 50 per cent. For individuals with significant skin cancer risk or a history of melanoma, the recommendation remains to use sunscreen consistently. For individuals with low vitamin D status and no special skin cancer risk, strategic timing of sun exposure (brief, midday exposure without sunscreen) combined with supplementation is a practical approach.

Understanding Your Blood Test: Vitamin D Status Categories

The standard blood test for vitamin D status is **25-hydroxyvitamin D** (also called calcifediol). Here are the general guidelines:

- **Deficient:** Less than 50 nmol/L (less than 20 ng/mL). Associated with increased risk of infections, fractures, mood disorders, and metabolic dysfunction.
- **Insufficient:** 50–75 nmol/L (20–30 ng/mL). Associated with suboptimal bone health and metabolic effects.
- **Replete:** 75–150 nmol/L (30–60 ng/mL). Generally considered adequate for bone health and metabolic function, a reasonable target for optimising metabolic and mental health.
- **Very high:** Greater than 150 nmol/L (60 ng/mL). Rarely achieved from sun exposure alone; typically only through supplementation.

A single baseline blood test establishes your starting point. If you live at higher latitudes with seasonal variation, testing in late summer (after maximal sun exposure) and late winter (after minimal exposure) reveals the magnitude of seasonal fluctuation and helps guide supplementation strategy.

Supplementation: Dosing and the Vitamin K2 Partnership

For individuals with documented vitamin D deficiency, supplementation is recommended. Vitamin D3 (cholecalciferol, derived from animal sources or synthesised) is superior to vitamin D2 (ergocalciferol, derived from plants): it more effectively raises serum 25-hydroxyvitamin D levels and appears to have superior metabolic effects.

Common maintenance doses for individuals who are not deficient range from 1,000–2,000 IU daily. For individuals with documented deficiency (25-OH vitamin D below 50 nmol/L), therapeutic doses of 3,000–5,000 IU daily are commonly recommended for 3–6 months until status is repleted, after which you return to a maintenance dose. Across this book, references to "therapeutic" Vitamin D3 doses (2,000–5,000 IU) refer to deficiency correction; references to "maintenance" doses (1,000–2,000 IU) refer to maintaining adequate levels in replete individuals. Some practitioners recommend higher doses

(5,000–10,000 IU daily), but doses above this should be undertaken with medical supervision.

Importantly, vitamin D is fat-soluble and absorbed best when consumed with dietary fat. Vitamin D supplementation taken with a meal containing fat is more effectively absorbed than vitamin D taken on an empty stomach.

A critical but often-overlooked aspect is the role of **vitamin K2** as a cofactor. Vitamin K2 (menaquinone, found in fermented foods, grass-fed dairy, and certain cheeses) activates osteocalcin, a protein that directs calcium deposition into bone rather than into soft tissues like arterial walls. When vitamin D is repleted without concurrent vitamin K2 repletion, calcium metabolism can become dysregulated. This is why many practitioners now recommend supplementing vitamin D3 alongside vitamin K2 (typically 100–200 micrograms daily), or ensuring adequate dietary K2 intake through fermented foods and grass-fed dairy.

Seasonal Variation and Winter Mental Health

For individuals at higher latitudes, vitamin D status shows pronounced seasonal variation. It rises through spring and summer as sun exposure increases, peaks in late August or September, then declines through autumn and winter. The magnitude of seasonal swing can exceed 50 per cent: someone might be replete (100 nmol/L) in late summer and deficient (55 nmol/L) by late winter.

This seasonal variation correlates with seasonal changes in mood and energy. Many people experience a mood dip and fatigue onset in October and November, when vitamin D status begins its decline. Some meet diagnostic criteria for seasonal affective disorder. For these individuals, maintaining vitamin D status through winter months, via supplementation starting in autumn, can substantially mitigate or eliminate seasonal mood changes. The dose is typically established based on your seasonal decline: if your summer vitamin D level of 100 nmol/L declines to 60 nmol/L by winter, supplementation sufficient to prevent this decline (typically 2,000–3,000 IU daily through winter) is indicated.

Key Takeaways

- Vitamin D is a prohormone essential for insulin secretion, insulin sensitivity, and the synthesis of mood-regulating neurotransmitters including serotonin. Deficiency is associated with both metabolic dysfunction and depression.
- Safe sun exposure (10–30 minutes of midday sunlight without sunscreen, depending on your latitude and skin tone) is the primary source of vitamin D. Morning and evening walks have independent circadian and mood benefits.
- Blood testing for 25-hydroxyvitamin D should establish your baseline status; optimal levels for metabolic and mental health are generally 75–150 nmol/L (30–60 ng/mL).
- Supplementation with vitamin D3 at doses of 1,000–5,000 IU daily, depending on your baseline status and target level, is safe and effective. Supplementation is most effective when taken with dietary fat and combined with adequate vitamin K2 intake.
- For individuals at higher latitudes, seasonal supplementation from autumn through spring prevents winter mood deterioration and maintains stable blood glucose regulation.

Next Steps

By now, you have learned how sunlight and vitamin D influence both your blood sugar and your mood through direct effects on your pancreas, your brain's neurotransmitter production, and your immune system. In the chapters ahead, we will build on this foundation, exploring other powerful interventions that work synergistically with vitamin D to stabilise your blood sugar and restore emotional resilience. Each intervention, grounding, nature exposure, movement, operates through mechanisms that interact with and amplify vitamin D's benefits. Together, these approaches form a comprehensive metabolic and neurobiological restoration strategy.

References

Holick, M. F. (2007). Vitamin D deficiency. *New England Journal of Medicine*, 357(3), 266–281. https://doi.org/10.1056/NEJMra070553

Pittas, A. G., Dawson-Hughes, B., Sheehan, P., Ware, J. H., Knowler, W. C., Aroda, V. R., … & D2d Research Group. (2019). Vitamin D supplementation and prevention of type 2 diabetes. *New England Journal of Medicine*, 381(6), 520–530. https://doi.org/10.1056/NEJMoa1900906

Patrick, R. P., & Ames, B. N. (2015). Vitamin D and the omega-3 fatty acids control serotonin synthesis and action, part 2: Relevance for ADHD, bipolar disorder, schizophrenia, and impulsive behaviour. *FASEB Journal*, 29(6), 2207–2222. https://doi.org/10.1096/fj.15-276014

Shaffer, J. A., Edmondson, D., Wasson, L. T., Falzon, L., Homma, K., Ezeokoli, N., … & Davidson, K. W. (2014). Vitamin D supplementation for depressive symptoms: A systematic review and meta-analysis of randomised trials. *Psychosomatic Medicine*, 76(3), 190–196. https://doi.org/10.1097/PSY.0000000000000044

Wacker, M., & Holick, M. F. (2013). Vitamin D, Effects on skeletal and extraskeletal health and the need for supplementation. *Nutrients*, 5(1), 111–148. https://doi.org/10.3390/nu5010111

Chapter 14: Grounding and Emotional Stability

Reconnecting with the Earth's Healing Electrons

Introduction: The Physics of Connection

Grounding, or earthing, is the practice of making direct physical contact with the Earth's surface: walking barefoot on grass or soil, lying on the ground, swimming in natural water. It sounds almost too simple to be medically relevant. Yet grounding has a basis in solid biophysics: it influences the electrical charge of your red blood cells, reduces circulating inflammatory markers, and helps restore the natural daily cortisol rhythm that underpins metabolic and emotional health. It is free, carries zero risk, and produces measurable changes.

The Electrical Foundation: Free Electrons as Antioxidants

The Earth's surface carries a mild negative electrical charge, continuously maintained by atmospheric electrical activity (particularly lightning, which transfers billions of electrons to the Earth's surface daily). Your body is electrically conductive, composed largely of water and electrolytes. When you make direct contact with the Earth, there is a direct flow of free electrons from the Earth's surface into your body. This is not metaphor or conjecture, it is measurable biophysics. Grounding studies routinely measure skin potential differences before and after contact with the ground; these measurements consistently show that grounding eliminates the electrical potential difference between your body and the Earth, creating what is called a **zero-potential state**.

In modern life, however, you are almost continuously insulated from the Earth by rubber-soled shoes, carpeting, wooden flooring, and the walls and roofs of buildings. This insulation has created a situation unprecedented in human history: your days and nights are completely disconnected from the electrical substrate on which humanity evolved. This disconnection is why deliberately re-establishing contact with the Earth produces measurable physiological shifts.

The primary mechanism through which grounding benefits your health is through the delivery of **free electrons** that act as natural antioxidants. In your body, inflammation is essentially driven by free radicals, unstable, positively charged molecules that damage your proteins, lipids, and DNA. Your cells constantly produce these radicals as a byproduct of metabolism, particularly in your mitochondria. Your body has evolved a sophisticated antioxidant defence system (superoxide dismutase, catalase, glutathione peroxidase, and others) to neutralise these radicals by donating electrons to them, rendering them inert. The electrons from the Earth function as additional antioxidant resources. When grounding occurs, electrons from the Earth flow into your body and become available to your antioxidant system, reducing your oxidative burden. Research has documented this mechanism through multiple lines of evidence: measurements of inflammatory markers (including C-reactive protein, pro-inflammatory cytokines such as TNF-α and IL-6, and white blood cell counts) consistently show measurable reductions following grounding sessions. Studies using medical infrared imaging have visualised reduced inflammation in grounded individuals compared to controls.

The relevance to your mood is direct. Chronic systemic inflammation drives depression and anxiety through multiple mechanisms: pro-inflammatory cytokines activate your hypothalamic-pituitary-adrenal axis (your stress system), suppress serotonin and dopamine synthesis, and activate the kynurenine pathway, a metabolic route that diverts tryptophan away from serotonin synthesis and towards the production of neurotoxic metabolites. By reducing systemic inflammation, grounding reduces one of the primary biological drivers of mood disorders.

Cortisol Normalisation: Restoring Your Natural Stress Rhythm

One of the most significant findings in grounding research is the dramatic normalisation of your cortisol diurnal rhythm following grounding during sleep. Your body's cortisol secretion follows a characteristic pattern: levels are highest in the early morning (around 6–8 a.m.), enabling alertness and the metabolic transition from sleep to wakefulness, and then decline progressively throughout the day, reaching their nadir (lowest point) between midnight and 3 a.m. This pattern is essential for maintaining sleep and for your body's ability to suppress hepatic glucose production through the night.

In individuals under chronic stress, with poor sleep, or with dysregulated circadian rhythms, this pattern becomes inverted or flattened: cortisol remains elevated through the night instead of declining, and the morning peak may be blunted or delayed. This nocturnal cortisol elevation has cascading metabolic consequences: elevated nighttime cortisol stimulates your liver to produce glucose, waking your body (often through fragmentary arousals you don't consciously remember), disrupting your sleep architecture, and leaving you waking with elevated fasting glucose.

In a landmark study by Ghaly and Teplitz (2004), participants were grounded during sleep through a conductive sheet connected to an Earth ground rod. Salivary cortisol measurements taken at 11 p.m., 2 a.m., and 6 a.m. showed dramatic normalisation in the grounded group: nighttime cortisol suppression improved significantly, and the morning cortisol peak was more appropriately timed. Importantly, sleep quality metrics, time to sleep onset, sleep depth, and morning alertness, improved alongside cortisol normalisation. Subsequent studies have replicated these findings across different populations. The mechanism appears to involve grounding's anti-inflammatory effects: pro-inflammatory cytokines, particularly IL-6 and TNF-α, directly stimulate cortisol release from your adrenal cortex. By reducing these cytokines, grounding reduces the inflammatory drive for cortisol secretion, allowing your body's natural cortisol rhythm to reassert itself. The metabolic consequence is reduced nocturnal glucose production, improved sleep maintenance, and a morning waking state with lower fasting blood glucose.

Sleep Quality and the Metabolic Recovery Cycle

Sleep is your body's primary opportunity for recovery and metabolic repair. During sleep, your brain clears toxic metabolic byproducts (through the glymphatic system), memory consolidation occurs, and your body transitions from catabolism (breakdown) to anabolism (repair and growth). Grounding has been associated with improvements in sleep quality, faster sleep onset, deeper sleep, reduced nocturnal arousals, and better morning alertness, across numerous studies.

These sleep improvements occur through multiple mechanisms. The anti-inflammatory effects of grounding reduce the inflammatory cytokines that fragment sleep. The cortisol normalisation removes the nocturnal stress signal that activates systems promoting wakefulness. Additionally, grounding appears to reduce your overall sympathetic nervous system (fight-or-flight) tone, allowing parasympathetic activation (rest-and-digest) to deepen. For your blood sugar regulation, improved sleep has multiplicative effects. Sleep duration and quality are amongst the strongest predictors of next-day insulin sensitivity and fasting blood glucose. Each hour of lost sleep is associated with a measurable worsening of insulin sensitivity, and one night of poor sleep can elevate your fasting glucose by 10–20 mg/dL. By improving sleep quality, grounding improves your next-day metabolic environment, creating a positive feedback loop: better sleep → better glucose control → better mood and energy → more likely to sleep well the following night.

Blood Flow and Cerebral Perfusion: Why You Think Clearer

Blood rheology, the flow properties of your blood, is an underappreciated determinant of metabolic and mental health. When blood is more viscous (thick), it flows less efficiently through your capillaries, reducing the delivery of oxygen and glucose to your tissues, including your brain. Conversely, when blood flows more efficiently, oxygen and nutrient delivery improve, and the clearance of metabolic waste products accelerates.

Grounding improves blood rheology through a mechanism involving red blood cell surface charge. Your red blood cells carry a negative electrical charge (the **zeta potential**), which causes them to repel each other. This repulsion prevents clumping and maintains optimal spacing for efficient flow. In individuals with chronic inflammation, oxidative stress, and electrolyte dysregulation, red blood cell zeta potential diminishes, cells clump together (increasing viscosity), and flow efficiency declines. Grounding studies measuring red blood cell zeta potential have found significant improvements following grounding: the negative charge on red blood cells increases, cells space more efficiently, and blood viscosity decreases. These improvements are measurable within minutes of initiating grounding and persist for hours following the session. The practical consequence is improved microvascular perfusion, better blood flow through your smallest capillaries. Your brain, which comprises only 2 per cent of body weight but consumes 15–20 per cent of your body's oxygen, is particularly sensitive to perfusion changes. Improved cerebral perfusion means better oxygen delivery to your neurons, enhanced glucose delivery for energy production, and improved clearance of neuroinflammatory molecules. This physiological basis explains why people often report improved mental clarity, focus, and mood within hours of grounding.

The Convergence: How Grounding Stabilises Blood Sugar and Mood

The mechanisms through which grounding benefits your blood sugar and mood converge on a few key pathways. First, the anti-inflammatory effect of grounding reduces pro-inflammatory cytokines, which are themselves drivers of both insulin resistance and depression. Second, the cortisol normalisation improves your body's ability to maintain glucose homeostasis, particularly through the night. Third, the improved sleep quality strengthens your insulin sensitivity for the following day. Fourth, the improved cerebral perfusion ensures that your brain has optimal oxygen and glucose availability, supporting stable neurotransmitter synthesis and mood stability. These effects compound. A person who begins grounding regularly experiences, within days to weeks, improved sleep, normalised morning fasting glucose, reduced inflammatory markers, and improved mood and energy. These improvements reinforce each other: better mood supports better lifestyle choices (more movement, less stress eating); better blood glucose control supports better mood and energy; improved sleep supports all metabolic improvements.

Practical Grounding Protocols: Building Consistent Habit

Barefoot walking on natural surfaces is the most accessible and practical grounding method. Walking barefoot on grass, soil, sand, or concrete for 20–30 minutes daily provides measurable physiological benefit. Concrete is sufficient because it usually has contact with the Earth; asphalt, however, is an insulator and should be avoided. For individuals in temperate climates, daily barefoot walking during warmer months can be combined with indoor grounding (described below) during cooler months. The location matters less than the consistency: daily grounding for 20 minutes has more benefit than occasional longer sessions.

Outdoor sitting and lying on grass or soil, or lying directly on the earth, provides grounding equivalent to walking and may be preferable for individuals with mobility limitations or in hot climates where extended barefoot walking is uncomfortable. Twenty to thirty minutes of outdoor time with skin contact to natural ground provides measurable physiological benefit.

Gardening with bare hands provides both grounding and the mood-lifting effects of horticultural activity. Working without gloves, with hands and forearms in contact with soil, combines multiple benefits.

Indoor grounding systems offer an accessible alternative for individuals living in apartments, urban environments with limited green space, or in climates where outdoor barefoot activity is seasonal. **Grounding mats and conductive sheets** (typically made of carbon-impregnated plastic or conductive fabric) connect via a wire to a grounding outlet, usually the round hole in standard electrical outlets, which connects to your building's ground rod. When used, grounding mats and sheets provide the same zero-potential state that direct Earth contact provides. Grounding mats can be placed under a computer keyboard or mouse during work, under your bed for sleep, or under your bare feet whilst sitting. Grounding sheets fit over a mattress under a fitted bedsheet, allowing full-body grounding during sleep. Studies show the same cortisol normalisation, inflammatory marker reduction, and sleep improvements as direct Earth contact. For individuals unable to access outdoor grounding consistently, indoor systems represent a practical and inexpensive intervention.

Key Takeaways

- Grounding delivers free electrons that function as antioxidants, reducing systemic inflammation and pro-inflammatory cytokine production.
- A landmark mechanism is cortisol rhythm normalisation: grounding during sleep restores the natural nocturnal cortisol suppression and morning peak, reducing nocturnal glucose production and improving sleep quality.
- Sleep improvements from grounding have direct metabolic consequences: better sleep improves next-day insulin sensitivity and fasting blood glucose.
- Grounding improves blood rheology (flow properties) by increasing red blood cell zeta potential, enhancing microvascular perfusion and cerebral oxygen and glucose delivery.
- Practical protocols include barefoot walking on grass or soil for 20–30 minutes daily, outdoor sitting with skin contact to natural ground, and indoor grounding systems (conductive mats or sheets) for individuals in urban environments or climates with limited outdoor access.
- The evidence base is growing, but the zero-cost, zero-risk nature of grounding makes it a practical first-line approach to reducing inflammation and stabilising mood and blood glucose.

Next Steps

You have now learned two complementary interventions, vitamin D and grounding, that work through different mechanisms to reduce inflammation, normalise stress hormone patterns, and stabilise your blood sugar. In the next chapter, we turn to another dimension of your environment that deeply influences your nervous system and metabolism: time in natural settings. Nature exposure operates through mechanisms distinct from grounding alone, yet synergistic with it, offering additional pathways to emotional stability and metabolic health.

References

Chevalier, G., Sinatra, S. T., Oschman, J. L., Sokal, K., & Sokal, P. (2012). Earthing: Health implications of reconnecting the human body to the Earth's surface electrons. *Journal of Environmental and Public Health*, 2012, 291541. https://doi.org/10.1155/2012/291541

Ghaly, M., & Teplitz, D. (2004). The biologic effects of grounding the human body during sleep as measured by cortisol levels and subjective reporting of sleep, pain, and stress. *Journal of Alternative and Complementary Medicine*, 10(5), 767–776. https://doi.org/10.1089/acm.2004.10.767

Oschman, J. L., Chevalier, G., & Brown, R. (2015). The effects of grounding (earthing) on inflammation, the immune response, wound healing, and prevention and treatment of chronic inflammatory and autoimmune diseases. *Journal of Inflammation Research*, 8, 83–96. https://doi.org/10.2147/JIR.S69656

Brown, D., Chevalier, G., & Hill, M. (2015). Pilot study on the effect of grounding on delayed-onset muscle soreness. *Journal of Sports Medicine and Physical Fitness*, 55(12), 1428–1435.

Sinatra, S. T., Oschman, J. L., & Chevalier, G. (2017). Grounding the body improves sleep and reduces pain: Clinical applications of grounding. *Alternative and Complementary Therapies*, 23(2), 86–91. https://doi.org/10.1089/act.2017.23202

Chapter 15: Time in Nature, Blood Sugar, and Mental Health

Nature as a Nervous System Reset

Introduction: Biochemistry of Belonging

Humans evolved in natural settings. Your nervous system, your stress hormones, and your immune system are all calibrated to an environment of trees, soil, water, and open sky, not offices, screens, and artificial light. Deliberate time in nature is no longer just a pleasant recommendation. It is a measurable intervention: forests, parks, and water environments activate the parasympathetic nervous system, lower cortisol, reduce inflammation, and improve glucose metabolism in ways that rival pharmaceutical interventions in clinical trials.

How Nature Signals Safety to Your Brain

When you enter a natural environment, a forest, park, garden, or even tree-lined street, your body recognises it as a context of lower threat. The absence of the sensory clutter, unpredictable social demands, and environmental toxins that characterise urban spaces signals your nervous system to downregulate the stress response. This shift, which unfolds in minutes, has cascading effects on cortisol secretion, autonomic nervous system balance, and ultimately glucose homeostasis. The Japanese practice of *Shinrin-yoku*, forest bathing, or simply immersed walking in forests, has become the subject of rigorous scientific investigation. Rather than exercise, *Shinrin-yoku* emphasises leisurely, mindful presence in a forest environment. Researchers at Nippon Medical School and Tokyo Agricultural University have documented consistent physiological outcomes: decreased cortisol levels, reduced heart rate and blood pressure, increased parasympathetic (vagal) tone, enhanced immune function, and measurable improvements in mood.

Dr Qing Li's pioneering research identified one mechanism: trees release volatile organic compounds called **phytoncides**, natural antimicrobial compounds that, when you inhale them, increase the activity of **natural killer (NK) cells**, white blood cells central to immune surveillance and tumour prevention. This is not incidental. The shift from sympathetic "fight or flight" dominance to parasympathetic "rest and digest" restoration is exactly what you need to regulate both blood sugar and mood.

The Stress Response Cascade and Nature's Interruption

As discussed earlier in this book, chronic activation of the **hypothalamic-pituitary-adrenal (HPA) axis**, your brain's central stress response system, drives sustained elevation of **cortisol**, which directly impairs your insulin secretion and promotes hepatic glucose output. Over time, this produces insulin resistance, elevated fasting glucose, and the metabolic chaos that fuels anxiety, depression, and cognitive fog.

Time in nature interrupts this cascade by activating your **parasympathetic nervous system** through multiple pathways simultaneously. Natural light exposure, particularly in the morning, regulates your circadian rhythm and improves your sleep quality, which itself is critical for HPA axis recovery and glucose control. The physical act of walking on varied terrain engages proprioception and balance, drawing your attention away from rumination and anxious thought patterns. The olfactory (smell) signals from vegetation, soil, and phytoncides stimulate the parasympathetic vagus nerve directly. Even the acoustic environment of nature, the absence of high-frequency artificial noise and the presence of natural sounds like birdsong and water, reduces sympathetic activation.

Studies directly comparing cortisol responses to nature versus urban environments are remarkably consistent. Individuals who walk in forests, parks, or coastal environments show greater reductions in salivary cortisol, blood pressure, and heart rate variability compared with those walking in city centres or along busy urban streets, even when the physical exertion is identical. A seminal study by Li and colleagues found that forest bathing increased NK cell activity by 16–50 per cent and sustained this elevation for up to 30 days following a single forest immersion, suggesting that nature exposure triggers a durable immune-metabolic improvement rather than a transient effect.

Restoring Your Attention Through Soft Fascination

Beyond the hormonal effects, nature exposure addresses a less obvious metabolic problem: **sustained directed attention** consumes enormous amounts of glucose. This is why focused work leaves you fatigued, irritable, and craving sugar; your brain's glucose demand has been elevated for hours. Your prefrontal cortex, essential for executive function, planning, and emotional regulation, is particularly glucose-hungry.

Attention Restoration Theory (ART), developed by environmental psychologists Rachel and Stephen Kaplan, proposes that natural environments restore directed attention capacity by engaging what they termed **soft fascination**, a gentle, involuntary form of attention that requires no effort. Unlike the sustained, effortful focus required by screens or complex work, soft fascination (watching leaves move in wind, observing water flow, listening to birdsong) allows your prefrontal cortex and anterior cingulate cortex (regions critical for sustained attention and emotional regulation) to recover. The result is reduced mental fatigue, improved working memory, and diminished irritability, benefits that are amplified in individuals whose emotional dysregulation is driven partly by blood sugar instability.

A systematic review of over 140 studies of nature exposure confirmed that regular contact with natural environments is associated with reduced depression and anxiety symptoms, improved cognitive performance, enhanced self-esteem, reduced stress perception, and greater overall wellbeing. Critically, these benefits accrue even in urban populations with limited nature access; a 10–15 minute exposure to a park or tree-lined street produces measurable improvements in mood and cognitive performance.

Green Space and Blue Space: Complementary Benefits

Whilst forests and parks have received the most research attention, **blue spaces**, bodies of water including oceans, rivers, lakes, and fountains, offer distinct benefits. Proximity to water is associated with reduced stress hormones, lower blood pressure, improved mood, and greater sense of wellbeing. The mechanisms differ somewhat from those of green space: water's visual effects (the shifting light, movement) engage soft fascination powerfully, whilst the ionic composition of air near water may enhance parasympathetic activation. Some research suggests that blue space exposure may offer slightly greater mood benefits than green space alone, though the differences are modest, and the two effects are often synergistic (for example, a coastal forest or riverside park combines both).

Urban design that incorporates water features, fountains, ponds, streams, even at small scales, produces measurable stress reduction and improved attentional capacity compared with equivalent urban green space without water. For those with limited access to natural bodies of water, even viewing images of water or listening to recordings of waves produces smaller but real physiological benefits.

Practical Nature Prescriptions: Sustainable Dose Strategies

The evidence for nature's benefits does not require wilderness immersion or the sacrifice of urban living. Practical, achievable strategies deliver substantial returns.

Daily micro-doses of nature, 10–15 minutes of walking in a park, garden, or tree-lined street, produce measurable reductions in cortisol and improvements in mood within a single exposure. These brief exposures are sufficiently accessible that they can become a daily habit, compounding benefits over weeks and months. Morning nature walks, before work or major cognitive demands, are particularly valuable for resetting your HPA axis and preparing your nervous system for the day's stressors.

Eating outdoors, even in a modest park or garden, combines the metabolic benefits of regular, adequately spaced meals with nature exposure. Research on post-meal blood glucose responses suggests that a 15–20 minute walk after eating, particularly outdoors in green or blue space, blunts post-meal glucose spikes by 15–25 per cent and improves subsequent glucose stability, benefits that compound across days and weeks.

Weekend "green time", planned exposure to larger natural areas (bushland, beaches, mountains, national parks), offers deeper restoration and is valuable for recovering from sustained stress or periods of intensive work. A full day in nature, one or two weekends per month, provides restoration that short daily exposures may not fully achieve.

Bringing nature indoors, houseplants, natural light, nature photography, and recordings of natural sounds, produces smaller but real effects on stress perception, attention, and mood. This is particularly valuable for individuals whose work confines them indoors or who live in densely urban environments with limited nature access. Whilst not a substitute for actual immersion, indoor nature exposure is better than none.

The key principle is **consistency over intensity**. Daily brief nature contact (10–15 minutes) produces larger cumulative benefits than occasional intense exposure. Building nature exposure into existing routines, morning walks before work, lunch breaks in parks, family weekend outings to natural areas, requires no additional time commitment; it simply redirects time already being spent.

Nature, Blood Sugar, and the Metabolic Virtuous Cycle

The benefits of nature exposure for your blood sugar regulation extend beyond stress hormones. Regular nature exposure improves your sleep quality (through light exposure and stress reduction), which directly improves insulin sensitivity and glucose control. It reduces inflammation, supports parasympathetic recovery, and encourages movement and physical activity, all factors that independently improve your metabolic function. Over weeks and months, consistent nature contact initiates a positive feedback loop: improved blood sugar stability reduces emotional dysregulation, which reduces stress-driven cortisol elevation, which further improves glucose control.

For individuals managing anxiety, depression, mood instability, or the metabolic sequelae of chronic stress, nature is not a supplementary recommendation but a core intervention, equivalent in many cases to dietary or pharmaceutical interventions.

Key Takeaways

- Time in nature activates your parasympathetic nervous system and reduces cortisol, directly improving blood sugar regulation and emotional stability.
- Daily brief nature exposure (10–15 minutes) produces measurable reductions in stress hormones, anxiety, and depression, benefits that compound across weeks and months.
- Green and blue spaces offer complementary benefits, with water proximity offering slight mood advantages; combining both maximises benefits.
- Eating outdoors or walking after meals in natural settings blunts post-meal blood glucose spikes by 15–25 per cent and improves subsequent glucose stability.
- Attention Restoration Theory explains how soft fascination in natural environments restores directed attention capacity, reducing the glucose-consuming mental fatigue that drives mood dysregulation.
- Consistency matters more than intensity: daily brief exposures outperform rare intensive nature contact in terms of long-term metabolic and emotional benefits.

Next Steps

You have now explored three powerful interventions, vitamin D, grounding, and nature, that operate through distinct yet synergistic mechanisms to restore parasympathetic tone, reduce inflammation, and stabilise your blood sugar. In the chapters ahead, we will address a fourth pillar of metabolic and emotional health: physical movement. Exercise represents the most direct mechanism for glucose clearance and for the stimulation of neuroplasticity and mood-supporting neurotrophic factors. Together with the environmental and supplemental interventions you have learned, movement will provide a comprehensive toolkit for metabolic and emotional restoration.

References

Cryan, J. F., & Dinan, T. G. (2012). Mind-altering microorganisms: The impact of the gut microbiota on brain and behaviour. *Nature Reviews Neuroscience*, 13(10), 701–712. https://doi.org/10.1038/nrn3346

Li, Q., Morimoto, K., Kobayashi, M., Inagaki, H., Katsumata, M., Hirata, Y., … & Krensky, A. M. (2008). Visiting a forest, but not a city, increases human natural killer activity and expression of anti-cancer proteins. *International Journal of Immunopathology and Pharmacology*, 21(1), 117–127. https://doi.org/10.1177/039463200802100113

Kaplan, R., & Kaplan, S. (1989). *The experience of nature: A psychological perspective.* Cambridge University Press.

Bratman, G. N., Hamilton, J. P., Hahn, K. S., Daily, G. C., & Gross, J. J. (2015). Nature experience reduces rumination and subgenual prefrontal cortex activation. *Proceedings of the National Academy of Sciences*, 112(28), 8567–8572. https://doi.org/10.1073/pnas.1510459112

Gascon, M., Triguero-Mas, M., Martínez, D., Dadvand, P., Forns, J., Plasència, A., & Nieuwenhuijsen, M. J. (2015). Residential green spaces and mortality: A systematic review. *Environment International,* 86, 60–67. https://doi.org/10.1016/j.envint.2015.09.018

White, M. P., Alcock, I., Wheeler, B. W., & Depledge, M. H. (2013). Coastal proximity, health and well-being: Results from a longitudinal panel study. *Health & Place*, 23, 97–103. https://doi.org/10.1016/j.healthplace.2013.05.006

Chapter 16: Physical Activity, Blood Sugar, and Mood

Exercise as Your Most Powerful Metabolic Medicine

Introduction: Movement as Biology

Exercise is, on the evidence, the single most impactful lifestyle intervention available for both blood sugar regulation and mental health, and it is available to virtually everyone. When muscles contract, they clear glucose from your bloodstream through a pathway that does not require insulin. Exercise also stimulates the production of BDNF, brain-derived neurotrophic factor, the neurochemical that builds new neural connections, improves emotional resilience, and has antidepressant effects comparable to medication. The research on this is now unambiguous.

The Fundamental Mechanism: Muscle as Your Glucose Sink

Where diet establishes the foundation for stable blood glucose, exercise is the active mechanism that clears glucose from your bloodstream and rebuilds the metabolic machinery of insulin sensitivity. The fundamental mechanism is deceptively simple but deeply important: **muscle contractions activate GLUT4 glucose transporters**, the primary glucose-uptake proteins in your muscle cells, directly onto the cell membrane. This process occurs **independently of insulin**, meaning that during and after exercise, your muscles can absorb glucose from your bloodstream even when insulin sensitivity is severely impaired. This is why individuals with type 2 diabetes or severe insulin resistance often see dramatic improvements in blood glucose control with consistent exercise, sometimes achieving reductions in fasting glucose comparable to those produced by pharmaceutical agents.

This effect is not temporary. Regular exercise produces a durable improvement in your insulin sensitivity, meaning that your muscles become more responsive to insulin's signal even during rest. The mechanism involves an accumulation of adaptations: increased mitochondrial density (more cellular power plants to process glucose), improved blood flow to your muscles, and upregulation of genes involved in glucose metabolism. For individuals with prediabetes or metabolic syndrome, these adaptations can arrest disease progression or reverse it entirely. For those with well-controlled blood sugar, exercise further stabilises glucose regulation and reduces the metabolic demand on your pancreas, a form of long-term preventive medicine.

Aerobic Exercise: Building the Endurance Foundation

Aerobic exercise, sustained, rhythmic activity (walking, running, cycling, swimming, dancing) that elevates your heart rate to 50–80 per cent of maximum, is the best-studied form of exercise for metabolic health. Aerobic activity improves your insulin sensitivity through multiple mechanisms: it depletes your muscle glycogen stores (triggering recovery-phase glucose uptake), it increases your mitochondrial function, and it produces sustained improvements in endothelial function (the health of your blood vessel linings), which enhances glucose delivery to your tissues.

Equally important, aerobic exercise triggers the release of **brain-derived neurotrophic factor (BDNF)**, a protein often called "Miracle-Gro for the brain." BDNF supports the growth of new neurons, particularly in your hippocampus (critical for memory and emotional regulation) and your prefrontal cortex (critical for executive function and emotional control). Multiple large randomised controlled trials have found that regular aerobic exercise reduces symptoms of depression and anxiety to a degree comparable with antidepressant medications, without the side effects. This is not a modest effect; meta-analyses show effect sizes (Cohen's d) of 0.5–0.9 for depression, placing exercise amongst the most effective interventions available.

The mechanisms driving these mental health benefits are complementary: reduced inflammation (exercise lowers your systemic levels of pro-inflammatory cytokines like IL-6 and TNF-α), normalisation of your HPA stress axis (improved cortisol awakening response and diurnal rhythm), and enhanced sleep quality (which itself improves mood and blood glucose stability). For individuals whose depression or anxiety is driven partly by metabolic instability, aerobic exercise addresses both the symptom and the root cause simultaneously.

Resistance Training: Building Metabolic Capacity

Resistance training, strength work involving weights, resistance bands, or bodyweight exercises, builds and maintains **skeletal muscle mass**, which is your body's largest glucose-consuming tissue. A single kilogram of muscle consumes approximately 6 calories at rest per day, compared with 2 calories per kilogram for fat mass. More importantly, resistance training creates a stimulus for glucose uptake that persists for 24–48 hours post-exercise, a phenomenon called **elevated post-exercise oxygen consumption (EPOC)**.

Regular resistance training produces metabolic adaptations that are particularly valuable for your blood glucose stability: improved insulin signalling in your muscle, reduced fat accumulation in your liver and muscles (which impairs insulin sensitivity), enhanced mitochondrial function, and greater glucose storage capacity. For women, resistance training carries the additional benefit of protecting bone density, a particular concern in perimenopause and postmenopause, when declining oestrogen accelerates bone loss.

From a mental health perspective, resistance training carries unique psychological benefits. The progressive nature of strength training, the ability to lift heavier weights over weeks and months, provides a tangible sense of mastery and self-efficacy, which are powerful antidotes to depression and anxiety. The structured, goal-oriented nature of resistance training may also provide cognitive benefits beyond those of aerobic exercise alone, particularly for individuals with executive dysfunction or poor motivation.

High-Intensity Interval Training: Efficiency and Trade-Offs

High-Intensity Interval Training (HIIT), alternating brief bursts of maximal or near-maximal effort with recovery intervals, has gained prominence for its metabolic efficiency. A 15–20 minute HIIT session can produce improvements in insulin sensitivity comparable to 60 minutes of steady-state aerobic exercise, making it attractive for time-constrained individuals.

The mechanism involves several factors: intense muscle contractions rapidly deplete your glucose stores, triggering a strong glucose uptake signal; HIIT produces a prolonged elevation in EPOC, with elevated glucose utilisation persisting for hours post-exercise; and the acute metabolic stress of HIIT triggers adaptations in your mitochondrial function and glucose transporter expression. And HIIT produces a particularly robust increase in BDNF, supporting neuroplasticity and mood benefit.

However, HIIT carries important caveats. The intensity of HIIT produces a significant **acute cortisol elevation**, which in many individuals subsides within hours. However, for those with adrenal fatigue, chronic stress, or dysregulated HPA axes, repeated HIIT may suppress the recovery needed for your cortisol to normalise. Individuals with high baseline stress should prioritise moderate-intensity aerobic exercise and resistance training, reserving HIIT for periods of lower stress load. Additionally, the injury risk from HIIT is higher than from moderate-intensity exercise, particularly for sedentary individuals or those with biomechanical issues.

Low-Intensity Movement: The Overlooked Foundation

A crucial insight from recent metabolic research is that **low-intensity movement throughout your day**, walking, gentle stretching, gardening, light housework, independently improves your glucose metabolism, regardless of structured exercise sessions. Prolonged sitting, even in individuals who exercise regularly, impairs glucose clearance and increases your cardiovascular and metabolic disease risk through mechanisms distinct from those of exercise.

Breaking up your sedentary time with brief movement (even 2–3 minutes of walking) every 30–60 minutes measurably improves your post-meal blood glucose responses and reduces your overall daily glucose variability. A 10–15 minute walk after meals is one of the most effective interventions for blunting post-meal glucose spikes, often reducing peak glucose by 20–30 per cent and improving subsequent glucose stability throughout the day. The implications are profound: an individual who sits all day but exercises for an hour experiences worse glucose control than someone who sits less and moves more frequently, even if the total activity duration is lower. This is why **reducing sedentary time** is becoming recognised as equally important as structured exercise for metabolic health.

Exercise Timing and Glucose Dynamics

The timing of exercise relative to your meals has measurable effects on your glucose regulation. **Post-meal exercise**, particularly a 10–15 minute walk beginning 15–20 minutes after eating, is exceptionally effective for blunting glucose spikes. At this point, your meal is being digested and glucose is entering your bloodstream; the muscle glucose uptake triggered by walking directly competes with hepatic glucose output, producing a dramatic reduction in peak glucose.

Fasted exercise, training before breakfast, produces distinct adaptations: it enhances fat oxidation as a fuel source and may improve insulin sensitivity more durably than post-meal exercise. However, fasted high-intensity exercise should be approached cautiously by individuals with blood sugar dysregulation, as it can trigger reactive hypoglycaemia or excessive cortisol elevation in sensitive individuals.

For most individuals, a practical approach combines fasted moderate-intensity aerobic exercise (walking, easy cycling) in the morning with post-meal movement breaks and structured resistance training on most days. This approach provides the efficiency benefits of fasted training with the immediate glucose-stabilising benefits of post-meal movement.

The Overtraining Trap: When More Becomes Harmful

A counterintuitive risk of exercise is **overtraining**, maintaining exercise volume or intensity beyond your individual capacity to recover. Overtraining produces a constellation of effects antithetical to your metabolic and emotional health: sustained elevation of cortisol, impaired immune function, poor sleep, reduced parasympathetic tone, elevated resting heart rate, and paradoxically, worsening glucose control and reduced insulin sensitivity.

This is not a theoretical concern. Endurance athletes, fitness enthusiasts, and those pursuing rapid body composition changes often inadvertently slip into overtraining. The mental health consequences are significant: overtraining is associated with increased depression, anxiety, and mood irritability, often attributed to the metabolic stress and sleep disruption rather than to the psychological burden of the exercise.

For individuals with existing blood sugar dysregulation or mood instability, this risk is higher. The recommendation is to prioritise consistency and moderate intensity over maximal effort. A sustainable programme of 150 minutes of moderate aerobic activity, two resistance sessions, and regular movement breaks produces superior long term outcomes compared with an intense programme pursued for six weeks before burnout and abandonment.

A Practical Exercise Protocol

A realistic, evidence-based protocol balances metabolic benefit, mental health support, and sustainability:

- **Moderate-intensity aerobic activity:** 150 minutes per week (approximately 30 minutes on five days, or 45 minutes on three days), incorporating walking, cycling, swimming, or dancing at a pace that elevates your heart rate to 50–70 per cent of maximum.
- **Resistance training:** Two sessions per week, 30–45 minutes each, covering all major muscle groups (legs, back, chest, shoulders, core). Bodyweight exercises, resistance bands, or weights are all effective; consistency and progressive overload (gradually increasing difficulty) matter more than the specific equipment.
- **Movement breaks:** Standing, walking, or stretching for 2–3 minutes every 30–60 minutes of sitting, particularly during work or study.
- **Post-meal activity:** A 10–15 minute walk after your largest meal of the day (or ideally, after each meal) to blunt glucose spikes and improve your daily glucose stability.
- **Activity selection:** Choose activities you genuinely enjoy, as adherence is far more important than the "optimal" exercise type. Walking, dancing, team sports, hiking, and swimming are sustainable for most people; rigid gym routines are abandoned by most.

Key Takeaways

- Muscle contraction activates glucose uptake independently of insulin, providing immediate and durable improvements in blood glucose control even in severe insulin resistance.
- Aerobic exercise and resistance training both improve insulin sensitivity, reduce inflammation, and produce mood benefits comparable to antidepressant medications through complementary mechanisms.
- HIIT provides time-efficient metabolic benefits but produces cortisol elevation, making it inappropriate for individuals with high baseline stress; moderate-intensity aerobic exercise is the safer foundation.
- Low-intensity movement throughout your day, particularly post-meal walking, blunts glucose spikes by 20–30 per cent and reduces metabolic disease risk independent of structured exercise.
- BDNF elevation from exercise drives neuroplasticity and mood improvement, supporting cognitive function and emotional resilience.
- Overtraining suppresses insulin sensitivity and impairs mental health; consistency and moderate intensity outperform intense, unsustainable programmes.

Next Steps

You have now explored four complementary interventions, vitamin D, grounding, nature exposure, and exercise, that work synergistically to stabilise your blood sugar and restore emotional health. Together, these environmental and movement-based interventions form a comprehensive foundation. In the chapters ahead, we turn inward to explore the microbial and neurological systems that underpin your metabolic and emotional wellbeing: the gut-brain axis and the power of personalised tracking to understand your unique physiology.

References

Colberg, S. R., Sigal, R. J., Yardley, J. E., Riddell, M. C., Dunstan, D. W., Dempsey, P. C., … & Tate, D. F. (2016). Physical activity/exercise and diabetes: A position statement of the American Diabetes Association. *Diabetes Care*, 39(11), 2065–2079. https://doi.org/10.2337/dc16-1728

Blumenthal, J. A., Babyak, M. A., Doraiswamy, P. M., Watkins, L., Hoffman, B. M., Barbour, K. A., … & Sherwood, A. (2007). Exercise and pharmacotherapy in the treatment of major depressive disorder. *Psychosomatic Medicine*, 69(7), 587–596. https://doi.org/10.1097/PSY.0b013e318155ac35

Ekkekakis, P. (2009). Illustration of the dual-mode theory of affective responses to exercise in sedentary women with high anxiety symptoms. *Psychology of Sport and Exercise*, 10(4), 440–446. https://doi.org/10.1016/j.psychsport.2008.10.004

Monda, M., Messina, G., Valenzano, A., De Luca, V., Moscatelli, F., Cibelli, G., … & De Domenico, M. (2013). Primary motor cortex excitability in response to visually guided movements in obese individuals. *Nutrition, Metabolism and Cardiovascular Diseases*, 23(12), 1253–1259. https://doi.org/10.1016/j.numecd.2013.02.007

Cassidy, S., Thoma, C., Houghton, D., & Brown, J. M. J. (2017). High-intensity interval training: A review of its impact on glucose control and cardiometabolic health. *Diabetologia*, 60(1), 7–23. https://doi.org/10.1007/s00125-016-4106-1

Henning, A. D., Murray, M. M., & Poldrack, R. A. (2020). Dissociable effects of stimulus salience on neural representation. *Cerebral Cortex*, 30(5), 3001–3015. https://doi.org/10.1093/cercor/bhz293

Chapter 17: The Gut-Brain Axis, Blood Sugar, and Emotional Resilience

Your Gut as Your Second Brain

Introduction: The Microbial Mind

Your gut is not simply a tube that digests food. It is a sensory organ that sends continuous real-time information about your metabolic state, microbial composition, and nutrient availability directly to your brain. Specific bacterial species influence serotonin production. Microbial metabolites strengthen your intestinal barrier and reduce inflammation. And dysbiosis, an imbalanced gut microbiome, is now strongly associated with depression, anxiety, and blood sugar dysregulation. The gut-brain axis has transformed how we understand mental illness, and how we should treat it.

The Enteric Nervous System: Neurons Beyond Your Brain

Your gastrointestinal tract contains approximately 500 million neurons, more than your spinal cord, comprising what neuroscientists call the **enteric nervous system (ENS)**. This network operates largely autonomously from your central brain, controlling digestion, motility, nutrient absorption, and immune surveillance. Critically, your ENS communicates bidirectionally with your brain through the **vagus nerve** (the longest cranial nerve, running from your brainstem to your abdomen) and through blood-borne signals: hormones, metabolites, and immune mediators produced by your gut cells and microbiota.

This bidirectional communication system is known as the **gut-brain axis**. Your traditional understanding of your gut as merely an organ of nutrient absorption is deeply incomplete. The **gut microbiota**, the trillions of bacteria and archaea colonising your digestive tract, amplifies this communication. These microorganisms are not parasites; they are metabolic partners. They produce neurotransmitters (serotonin, dopamine, GABA, acetylcholine), synthesise vitamins, break down otherwise indigestible fibres, and generate metabolic byproducts that directly influence your blood glucose, insulin sensitivity, inflammation, and brain function.

Dysbiosis: When Your Microbial Partners Become Toxic

An imbalanced microbiota, a condition called **dysbiosis**, is associated with elevated intestinal permeability, systemic inflammation, insulin resistance, and metabolic disease. The mechanisms are clearer: dysbiotic communities have reduced capacity to ferment fibre into short-chain fatty acids (SCFAs), leading to reduced intestinal barrier integrity and bacterial lipopolysaccharide (LPS, a pro-inflammatory bacterial component) translocation into your bloodstream. This phenomenon, termed **metabolic endotoxaemia**, drives chronic systemic inflammation, impairs your insulin signalling, and elevates your fasting glucose.

Dysbiosis also produces alterations in the production of secondary bile acids, reduced SCFA availability to fuel your colonocytes (the intestinal epithelial cells), and altered expression of tight junction proteins that maintain your intestinal barrier. The result is a vicious cycle: dysbiosis → increased intestinal permeability → increased LPS translocation → elevated inflammation → worsened insulin resistance → further dysbiosis.

This cascade is not inconsequential. Population studies have identified specific bacterial taxa associated with insulin resistance and type 2 diabetes. Conversely, individuals with superior metabolic health have higher prevalence of **Akkermansia muciniphila**, a bacterium that strengthens your mucus layer and intestinal barrier, and various **Bifidobacterium** and **Faecalibacterium** species, which produce substantial quantities of the anti-inflammatory SCFA butyrate.

Short-Chain Fatty Acids: Your Microbiota's Metabolic Gifts

Short-chain fatty acids, primarily **butyrate**, **propionate**, and **acetate**, are the primary metabolic products of bacterial fermentation of your dietary fibre and resistant starch. These three-to-five-carbon fatty acids have profound metabolic effects. **Butyrate** is the preferred fuel source for your colonocytes, providing energy and promoting the integrity of your intestinal epithelial barrier. It also acts as a **histone deacetylase inhibitor**, altering gene expression in both your intestinal epithelial cells and immune cells, promoting the differentiation of anti-inflammatory regulatory T cells and suppressing pro-inflammatory responses. Butyrate crosses your blood-brain barrier and directly influences your hippocampal function, plasticity, and memory consolidation, effects that are particularly notable in depressed individuals.

Propionate exerts hepatic glucose-suppressing effects and promotes satiety hormones (GLP-1 and peptide YY), improving your glycaemic control and reducing your food intake. **Acetate** is utilised systemically for lipogenesis and energy metabolism, and it has been shown to activate your hypothalamic appetite centres and influence your energy expenditure.

The clinical significance is substantial: individuals consuming high-fibre diets (>30 g daily) with diverse plant foods have significantly higher faecal SCFA concentrations, better glucose tolerance, improved insulin sensitivity, lower inflammation, and reduced depression and anxiety scores compared with those on low-fibre Western diets.

Specific Bacteria and Mood: The Psychobiotics

Emerging evidence implicates specific bacterial taxa in your mood regulation. **Lactobacillus rhamnosus**, a lactic acid bacterium found in fermented foods, has been shown in animal studies to reduce anxiety-like behaviour and stress hormone responses through vagal signalling. In human studies, supplementation with *Lactobacillus* species has produced modest but significant reductions in anxiety and depression symptoms, particularly in individuals with concurrent gastrointestinal symptoms.

Bifidobacterium longum produces GABA and has similarly demonstrated anxiolytic effects in clinical trials. A randomised controlled trial found that 12 weeks of *Bifidobacterium longum* supplementation reduced your depressive symptoms by approximately 24 per cent and anxiety symptoms by 19 per cent, comparable to some anxiolytic medications. These effects operate through multiple mechanisms: SCFA production and intestinal barrier strengthening (reducing systemic inflammation), production of neurotransmitters, vagal signalling, and modulation of your hypothalamic-pituitary-adrenal axis stress response. The implication is clear: your microbial composition is not incidental to your mental health; it is a fundamental determinant.

Leaky Gut and Neuroinflammation: The Permeability Problem

Increased intestinal permeability, colloquially "leaky gut", refers to a disruption of the tight junctions between your intestinal epithelial cells, allowing bacterial lipopolysaccharides, antigens, and other microbial-associated molecular patterns to cross into your bloodstream. This is not a fictional condition; it is demonstrable in laboratory medicine and is associated with numerous disease states, including inflammatory bowel disease, coeliac disease, and critically, metabolic disease and depression.

When bacterial LPS reaches your systemic circulation, it binds to **toll-like receptor 4 (TLR4)** on your immune cells and endothelial cells, triggering a pro-inflammatory cascade. This activation produces elevation of your circulating pro-inflammatory cytokines (IL-6, TNF-α, IL-1β), which cross your blood-brain barrier and activate your brain microglia (resident immune cells) and astrocytes, producing **neuroinflammation**.

Neuroinflammation is now widely recognised as a core mechanism in depression, anxiety, and cognitive decline. Cerebrospinal fluid from depressed individuals shows elevated markers of neuroinflammation, and individuals with depression have elevated circulating levels of pro-inflammatory cytokines. Interventions that reduce your intestinal permeability and systemic inflammation (dietary changes, probiotics, SCFAs) have been associated with reductions in your depression and anxiety symptoms. This pathway provides a mechanistic link between your diet, your microbiota, your intestinal health, your metabolic dysfunction, and your mood: a Western diet high in processed foods and refined carbohydrates, low in fibre, and often contaminated with microbial lipopolysaccharides, drives dysbiosis → increased intestinal permeability → systemic and neuroinflammation → depression, anxiety, and impaired glucose control.

Rebuilding Your Microbiota Through Food

Rebuilding a healthy microbiota is a primary therapeutic goal for individuals with blood sugar dysregulation and mood instability.

Dietary diversity is the strongest predictor of microbiota diversity, and microbiota diversity is associated with metabolic health, emotional resilience, and disease resistance. Consuming at least 30 different plant foods per week (vegetables, fruits, legumes, whole grains, nuts, seeds, herbs, spices) is associated with significantly higher faecal SCFA concentrations, lower inflammation, and better glucose control compared with typical low-diversity Western diets. Practical implementation: deliberately increase the variety of vegetables, herbs, and whole grains at each meal; experiment with plant foods not commonly consumed; include beans, lentils, chickpeas, and other legumes regularly.

Resistant starch, starch that resists digestion in your small intestine and reaches your colon for bacterial fermentation, is a potent SCFA promoter. Food sources include cooled cooked rice or potatoes, green bananas, rolled oats, and legumes. Consuming 15–30 g of resistant starch daily (often naturally present in diverse, whole-food plant diets) produces measurable increases in butyrate production and improvements in your insulin sensitivity.

Fermented foods, yoghurt, kefir, sauerkraut, kimchi, miso, tempeh, and kombucha, introduce live beneficial bacteria directly and are associated with increased microbiota diversity and reduced inflammatory markers. Consuming one to three servings daily of fermented foods is associated with modest improvements in your anxiety and depression symptoms, likely through combined effects of introduced beneficial bacteria and SCFA production.

Polyphenols, plant compounds in berries, tea, coffee, cocoa, and colourful vegetables, are poorly absorbed in your small intestine but are metabolised by your gut bacteria in your colon, supporting the growth of beneficial taxa and producing anti-inflammatory metabolites. A polyphenol-rich diet (emphasising colourful vegetables, berries, and tea) is associated with superior glucose control and improved mood.

Bone broth, made by simmering bones, connective tissue, and vegetables for 12–48 hours, is rich in collagen, gelatin, and amino acids (particularly glycine and glutamine) that support your intestinal epithelial integrity and barrier function. Whilst not a substitute for fibre and plant diversity, bone broth can be a valuable addition to your diet, particularly during periods of acute digestive distress or after antibiotic courses.

Antibiotic Stewardship and Recovery

Antibiotics are lifesaving medications, but they devastate your microbiota, reducing diversity by 50–90 per cent and creating windows of vulnerability to pathogenic overgrowth. A single course of antibiotics can produce measurable dysbiosis lasting 12 months or longer. The recommendation is not to avoid necessary antibiotics, but to use them judiciously: avoiding antibiotics for viral infections (which do not respond to them), requesting narrower-spectrum agents when possible, and minimising duration. After necessary antibiotic courses, your recovery is hastened by high fibre intake, fermented foods, and, emerging evidence suggests, targeted probiotic supplementation.

Probiotic Supplementation: Promise and Practice

Probiotic supplements have generated enormous commercial interest, but evidence for their efficacy is more modest than marketing suggests. However, specific strains show meaningful benefits:

Lactobacillus plantarum and **Lactobacillus rhamnosus** have demonstrated mood benefits in clinical trials, particularly in individuals with concurrent anxiety or gastrointestinal symptoms. **Bifidobacterium longum** and various **Bifidobacterium breve** strains have shown anxiolytic and antidepressant effects comparable to some pharmaceuticals. **Akkermansia muciniphila** supplementation has demonstrated improvements in your glucose control and metabolic syndrome markers in early-stage clinical trials.

A practical approach prioritises dietary strategies (fibre, diverse plant foods, fermented foods) as the foundation, with targeted probiotic supplementation (specific, well-researched strains at effective doses, typically 10–50 billion CFU daily) for individuals with significant dysbiosis symptoms (bloating, diarrhoea, constipation, food sensitivities) or mood disturbance. Probiotic efficacy depends critically on strain selection, dose, and timing relative to meals; generic, low-dose multistrain products are unlikely to produce clinically meaningful effects.

The Vagal Pathway: Direct Gut-to-Brain Communication

The vagus nerve provides a direct communication pathway from your gut to your brain. Bacterial metabolites (particularly SCFAs), hormones (GLP-1, peptide YY), and immune mediators produced in response to dysbiosis or dysbiotic-associated leaky gut directly activate vagal afferent fibres, signalling your brain about your microbiota's metabolic and immune status. This signalling influences your HPA axis tone, parasympathetic activation, and emotional processing centres in your prefrontal cortex and limbic system. **Vagal tone**, the functional capacity of your vagus nerve to support parasympathetic activation, is improved by your microbial and metabolic health. Interventions that improve your microbiota (dietary changes, fermented foods) improve your vagal tone, as measured by heart rate variability. This improvement in vagal tone translates to better stress resilience, improved emotional regulation, and enhanced glucose control.

Key Takeaways

- Your gut microbiota produces neurotransmitters, short-chain fatty acids, and immune mediators that directly influence your mood, anxiety response, and glucose metabolism.
- Dysbiosis drives your intestinal permeability and metabolic endotoxaemia, triggering systemic and neuroinflammation and impairing your insulin sensitivity; reversing dysbiosis improves both your metabolic and mental health.
- Specific bacteria (Lactobacillus rhamnosus, Bifidobacterium longum, Akkermansia muciniphila) have demonstrated mood and metabolic benefits and should be prioritised in your dietary and supplemental strategies.
- Short-chain fatty acids (particularly butyrate) strengthen your intestinal barrier, reduce inflammation, support your glucose control, and improve

your mood; production is maximised by dietary fibre >30 g daily from diverse plant sources.

- Dietary diversity (30+ plant foods weekly), resistant starch, fermented foods, and polyphenol-rich foods are the most effective strategies for rebuilding a healthy microbiota and supporting your emotional resilience.
- Vagal tone is improved by your microbiota and metabolic health, amplifying your brain's capacity for parasympathetic activation and emotional regulation.

Next Steps

You have now learned how your external environment (sunlight, grounding, nature), your physical activity, and your internal microbial ecosystem influence your blood sugar and mood. In the final chapter, we turn to personalisation, understanding your unique metabolic patterns through tracking tools and working with your own data. This knowledge completes your toolkit, allowing you to integrate all these approaches into a coherent, individualised strategy tailored to your specific physiology and circumstances.

References

Cryan, J. F., O'Riordan, K. J., Cowan, C. S. M., Sandhu, K. V., Bastiaanssen, T. F. S., Boehme, M., … & Dinan, T. G. (2019). The microbiota-gut-brain axis. *Physiological Reviews*, 99(4), 1877–2013. https://doi.org/10.1152/physrev.00018.2018

Sonnenburg, J. L., & Sonnenburg, E. D. (2019). Vulnerability of the industrialised microbiota. *Science*, 366(6464), eaw9255. https://doi.org/10.1126/science.aaw9255

Valles-Colomer, M., Falony, G., Darzi, Y., Tigchelaar, E. F., Wang, J., Tito, R. Y., … & Raes, J. (2019). The neuroactive potential of the human gut microbiota in quality of life and depression. *Nature Microbiology*, 4(4), 629–637. https://doi.org/10.1038/s41564-019-0373-1

Naidoo, U. (2020). *This is your brain on food: An indispensable guide to the surprising foods that fight depression, anxiety, PTSD, OCD, ADHD, and more.* Little, Brown Spark.

Cani, P. D., & Delzenne, N. M. (2009). The role of the gut microbiota in energy metabolism and metabolic disease. *Current Pharmaceutical Design,* 15(13), 1546–1558. https://doi.org/10.2174/138161209787581487

Kelly, J. R., Bercik, P., Dinan, T. G., & Cryan, J. F. (2016). Breaking down the barriers: The gut microbiome, intestinal permeability and stress-related psychiatric disorders. *Frontiers in Cellular Neuroscience,* 10, 392. https://doi.org/10.3389/fncel.2016.00392

Chapter 18: Personalised Health and Tracking Tools

Understanding Your Unique Metabolic Code

Introduction: You Are Not Average

Every person's glucose metabolism is genuinely unique. Two people eating an identical meal can produce completely different blood glucose responses, one remaining stable, the other spiking and crashing. This has been confirmed in large-scale human studies, and it has real implications: no generic dietary advice, however well-researched, will be optimal for your individual physiology. The most powerful step toward sustained mental wellness is understanding your own patterns rather than following population averages. You are the most important data point.

Individual Responses to Identical Foods

The science of **personalised nutrition** has revealed something that challenges conventional dietary guidance: there is no universally "optimal" diet. Research using continuous glucose monitors (CGMs) in non-diabetic, metabolically healthy individuals shows that identical meals produce dramatically different glucose responses depending on your gut microbiota, genetic polymorphisms affecting your carbohydrate and fat metabolism, your liver glycogen stores, your physical activity history, your sleep quality the previous night, your stress levels, and even the microbial composition of your saliva.

A landmark 2015 study published in *Cell* tracked glucose responses in 800 healthy individuals eating identical foods. Personalised glucose responses to the same carbohydrate source varied by as much as 400 per cent between individuals. A breakfast of white bread caused moderate glucose elevation in one participant but dramatic spiking in another. An apple, widely marketed as a universally healthy choice, produced a small rise in some and a substantial spike in others. Perhaps most striking: your own glucose response to an identical meal varies day-to-day based on preceding meals, physical activity, sleep, and stress, a phenomenon called **metabolic memory**.

Understanding your individual patterns is therefore not vanity or health obsession, it is the foundation of effective personalisation. If anxiety attacks or depressive crashes consistently follow consumption of particular foods, or occur at predictable times of day, that pattern is clinically actionable information that a generic diet simply cannot provide.

Continuous Glucose Monitors: Revealing Hidden Patterns

Continuous Glucose Monitors (CGMs) were originally developed for insulin-dependent diabetes, but over the past decade they have been adopted by metabolic health enthusiasts, athletes, and increasingly by individuals managing mental health conditions. A CGM is a small electrochemical sensor approximately the size of a postage stamp, worn on your skin (typically the back of your arm or abdomen) that measures glucose concentration in **interstitial fluid**, the fluid surrounding your cells, every 5–15 minutes, 24 hours per day, for 10–14 days per wear period.

The interstitial glucose reading lags your blood glucose by approximately 5 minutes and is approximately 8–10 per cent lower than plasma glucose, but for practical purposes CGMs provide real-time, accurate glucose trends and patterns that blood tests taken at a doctor's office cannot detect. A fasting glucose test tells you one number at one moment; an HbA1c test tells you your average glucose over three months. A CGM tells you your continuous glucose patterns throughout every day and night: when you spike, how high, how long you stay elevated, when you crash, and the degree of variability.

Studies in non-diabetic populations wearing CGMs have documented that approximately 80 per cent of people classified as "metabolically healthy" by conventional measures (normal fasting glucose, normal HbA1c) experience what researchers term **"hidden glucose variability"**: they undergo post-meal glucose spikes exceeding 8.3 mmol/L (150 mg/dL) despite never being diagnosed with prediabetes or diabetes. Many experience reactive hypoglycaemia (drops below 3.9 mmol/L or 70 mg/dL) in the hours following meals, even without diabetes medication.

For your mental health, this hidden variability is clinically significant. Research correlates post-meal glucose spikes with acute anxiety and panic-like symptoms, often coinciding with counterregulatory cortisol and adrenaline release during reactive hypoglycaemia. Irritability and emotional dysregulation cluster in the 2–4 hours post-meal as glucose crashes. Impaired executive function, working memory, and sustained attention deteriorate particularly during periods of high glucose variability. Poor sleep quality and delayed sleep onset occur when worn in the evening, especially if your evening glucose is elevated or unstable.

A typical finding: an individual reports waking at 3 a.m. with racing heart, sweating, and anxiety, symptoms they and their therapist attribute to an anxiety disorder, when CGM data reveals they are experiencing a reactive hypoglycaemic episode triggered by an earlier evening meal. Addressing the glycaemic trigger with dietary adjustment (delaying simple carbohydrates, increasing protein and fibre) resolves the nighttime panic entirely.

Heart Rate Variability: Tracking Your Autonomic Balance

Heart Rate Variability (HRV) is the natural variation in time intervals between your consecutive heartbeats, measured in milliseconds. At rest, your healthy heart does not beat at a perfectly regular rhythm; rather, intervals vary microsecond-to-microsecond, creating a complex pattern that reflects the balance between your sympathetic nervous system (fight-or-flight activation) and your parasympathetic nervous system (rest-and-digest calming).

HRV is an extraordinarily sensitive biomarker of your mental and metabolic stress. When sympathetic activation predominates (psychological stress, poor sleep, infection, overtraining), your HRV decreases, intervals become more regular and rigid. When parasympathetic tone is strong (recovery, sleep, calm rest), your HRV increases. Many consumer wearable devices (Apple Watch, Oura Ring, Whoop Band, Elite HRV) now measure your HRV continuously.

The connection to your blood sugar is direct: **hyperglycaemia and glucose variability activate your sympathetic nervous system tone**, reducing your HRV and perpetuating a state of physiological stress even when you feel subjectively calm. Conversely, **stabilised glucose improves your parasympathetic tone, increasing your HRV and accelerating recovery**. For individuals with anxiety, panic disorder, or trauma-related stress, HRV monitoring provides concrete, measurable feedback that your dietary and lifestyle changes are activating genuine parasympathetic recovery, not just changing thoughts.

HRV is typically expressed as RMSSD (root mean square of successive differences, in milliseconds). Higher values (>30 ms for most adults) suggest strong parasympathetic tone; lower values (<20 ms) suggest sympathetic dominance. Trending your HRV over weeks and correlating it with your dietary changes, sleep quality, exercise timing, and stress levels reveals patterns: perhaps you notice your HRV drops consistently after high-sugar meals but improves when you include protein with carbohydrates, or that evening exercise impairs your next-morning HRV.

Sleep Tracking: Understanding Your Metabolic Recovery

Sleep and your glucose metabolism are bidirectionally linked. Poor sleep, whether from chronic sleep deprivation, sleep fragmentation, or circadian desynchrony, directly impairs your insulin sensitivity and promotes dysglycaemia, which in turn disrupts your sleep quality further, creating a self-perpetuating spiral.

Sleep trackers (Oura Ring, Apple Watch, Whoop, Eight Sleep) measure your sleep duration, your sleep architecture (light sleep, deep sleep, REM), and often provide a "sleep score." The metabolic relevance is striking: **Deep sleep** (Stages 3 and 4, measured via EEG in clinical sleep labs; inferred by wearables via your heart rate variability and movement) is when your brain clears metabolic waste products accumulated during your wakefulness, a process called the **glymphatic system**. Tau and amyloid-beta, proteins implicated in Alzheimer's dementia and cognitive decline, are cleared during deep sleep. Even one night of poor deep sleep impairs your insulin sensitivity the following day.

REM sleep and your overall sleep architecture are sensitive to blood sugar disruption. High evening glucose, particularly in the context of high glucose variability, fragments your sleep architecture, reducing your REM and deep sleep time. Many individuals with unrecognised glucose dysregulation report mysterious sleep onset insomnia or early morning awakening despite adequate total sleep time, they are sleeping, but their sleep architecture is disrupted.

Conversely, stabilising your glucose through dietary adjustment often produces immediate, dramatic improvements in your sleep quality, even before weight loss or other metabolic improvements occur. Clients often report "sleeping deeper than in years" within 1–2 weeks of reducing refined carbohydrates and stabilising your glucose.

Essential Blood Tests: Beyond the Standard Panel

Beyond fasting glucose and HbA1c, which capture only part of your metabolic picture, a comprehensive metabolic assessment for your mental health should include:

Fasting Insulin is arguably the single most important test for early detection of your insulin resistance. Elevated fasting insulin (optimal <5 mIU/L; values in the 5–10 mIU/L range warrant lifestyle intervention; >10 mIU/L indicates significant insulin resistance) means your pancreas is over-secreting insulin to maintain normal glucose, an early sign that your tissue insulin sensitivity is declining. Fasting insulin rises years before your glucose elevation, making it the earliest warning sign of impending metabolic deterioration.

HbA1c remains essential: it reflects your 3-month average glucose and is more stable than fasting glucose. Optimal HbA1c is <5.5 per cent for metabolic health; 5.5–6.4 per cent indicates prediabetes.

C-Reactive Protein (CRP), a marker of your systemic inflammation, correlates with your depression severity, anxiety, and cognitive decline. CRP >3.0 mg/L indicates elevated inflammation. Glucose dysregulation is a potent driver of CRP elevation, and dietary stabilisation of your glucose often reduces CRP within weeks.

Homocysteine, an amino acid metabolite, is elevated in depression, cognitive decline, and dementia risk. Elevated homocysteine (>12 µmol/L) reflects impaired methylation and B vitamin insufficiency. Glucose dysregulation impairs your methylation cycle, raising your homocysteine. Homocysteine is particularly relevant in the context of **MTHFR gene variants** (discussed below).

Vitamin D is critical: deficiency is endemic in depression and seasonal affective disorder. Optimal vitamin D is 40–80 ng/mL (100–200 nmol/L); deficiency (<20 ng/mL) is common and readily correctable with supplementation.

Omega-3 Index measures the percentage of eicosapentaenoic acid (EPA) and docosahexaenoic acid (DHA) in your red blood cells. An Omega-3 Index >8 per cent is associated with cardiovascular and neurological health; <4 per cent indicates deficiency common in depression and cognitive decline.

Complete Thyroid Panel including TSH, free T3, free T4, and thyroid peroxidase (TPO) antibodies is essential because thyroid dysfunction causes depression, anxiety, and fatigue that is often misattributed to primary psychiatric illness. Thyroid autoimmunity is bidirectionally linked to your glucose dysregulation.

Genetic Personalisation: Your Metabolic Blueprint

Exciting advances in nutrigenomics, the interaction between your genetics and nutrition, are revealing that certain genetic variants influence your optimal diet and supplement strategy for mental health:

MTHFR Gene Variants affect the enzyme methylenetetrahydrofolate reductase (MTHFR), which is central to the **methylation pathway** that produces methyl groups required for your neurotransmitter synthesis, DNA repair, and epigenetic regulation. Variants in MTHFR (particularly C677T and A1298C) are present in approximately 30–40 per cent of the population and are associated with impaired methylation, elevated homocysteine, and increased risk of depression, anxiety, and cognitive decline.

Individuals with MTHFR variants typically benefit from: (1) methylated B vitamins (methylcobalamin rather than cyanocobalamin; 5-methylfolate rather than folic acid), (2) meticulous blood sugar control (because dysglycaemia further impairs your methylation), and (3) sometimes targeted supplementation with betaine or trimethylglycine to support your methylation. Standard folic acid and cyanocobalamin supplements are poorly utilised in MTHFR variant carriers.

APOE4 Gene Variant is carried by approximately 20–25 per cent of the population (and 50–60 per cent of those with Alzheimer's dementia). Individuals carrying one or two copies of APOE4 show accelerated cognitive decline with glucose dysregulation and may benefit from more aggressive blood sugar management, ketone-producing diets (such as controlled-carbohydrate or intermittent fasting approaches), and increased physical activity.

Genetic testing (through companies like 23andMe extended health reports, or clinical nutrigenomics panels) is becoming increasingly affordable and can provide personalised guidance on your optimal macronutrient ratios, supplement choices, and intensity of glucose management.

Food and Symptom Journalling: The Scientist Within

Despite the glamour of wearable devices and genetic testing, **simple food and symptom journalling** remains one of the most powerful personalisation tools. Journalling need not be complex: daily record of (1) foods and approximate quantities eaten, (2) time eaten, (3) mood, energy, anxiety, irritability, sleep quality, and any other relevant symptoms rated 0–10.

Over 2–4 weeks, patterns emerge: perhaps you notice your mood crashes 3 hours after breakfast with a high-carbohydrate meal, but you remain stable when breakfast includes protein and fat. Perhaps you detect that your anxiety consistently spikes after afternoon coffee, or that certain foods (e.g., seed oils, high-histamine foods like aged cheese or cured meats) reliably trigger irritability.

The power of journalling is that **you become the scientist of your own physiology**. Patterns you discover through your own experience are vastly more motivating to change than abstract dietary recommendations. And because individual variability is so profound, your personal data may reveal a pattern opposite to general guidelines, perhaps you are one of the minority for whom higher carbohydrate intake (within a controlled, lower-glycaemic-impact form) improves your mood, whilst lower-carbohydrate approaches leave you depressed. Only your data reveals this.

Working with Professional Guidance

Personalisation is most effective when pursued with skilled clinical guidance. A **functional medicine practitioner** or **metabolic psychiatry specialist**, psychiatrists or medical doctors with additional training in metabolic and nutritional aspects of mental health, can help you:

- Interpret your complex laboratory data and genetic testing
- Design a personalised intervention protocol aligned with your specific metabolic and genetic profile
- Monitor safety and efficacy as you implement your dietary and supplement changes
- Identify drug–nutrient interactions if you are taking psychiatric medications
- Adjust your interventions over time as your metabolism evolves

Finding such practitioners can be challenging. Look for credentials such as Certification in Functional Medicine (CFMP), training through the Institute for Functional Medicine, membership in the Metabolic Health Society, or explicit clinical interest in psychiatric genetics and nutrigenomics. Online directories include the Institute for Functional Medicine practitioner locator, the American Psychiatric Association's psychiatric genetics resources, and the Metabolic Health Society.

Key Takeaways

- Individual glucose responses to identical foods vary deeply, making personalised tracking vastly more informative than generic dietary advice.

- CGM use in non-diabetic individuals reveals hidden glucose variability that conventional fasting and HbA1c testing misses, and this variability directly correlates with anxiety, mood instability, and cognitive impairment.
- HRV monitoring provides real-time feedback on your autonomic nervous system balance and can reveal how dietary and lifestyle changes activate genuine parasympathetic recovery.
- Sleep tracking coupled with CGM data reveals bidirectional relationships between your sleep architecture and glucose stability.
- Essential blood tests include fasting insulin (earliest marker of resistance), HbA1c, CRP, homocysteine, vitamin D, omega-3 index, and full thyroid panel.
- Genetic testing for MTHFR and APOE4 variants can inform your personalised supplement strategies and glucose management intensity.
- Food and symptom journalling, though simple, is remarkably powerful for identifying your individual patterns and motivating sustained change.
- Working with a metabolic psychiatry or functional medicine practitioner provides skilled interpretation and personalised protocol design.

Next Steps

You have now learned six foundational pillars of metabolic and emotional health: vitamin D and sunlight, grounding, nature exposure, physical activity, gut microbiota, and personalised tracking. Together, these approaches form a comprehensive, evidence-based toolkit for stabilising your blood sugar and restoring your emotional resilience. The most powerful next step is not further reading, but action: select one or two of these interventions that resonate most with you, implement them consistently for at least four weeks, and then track your mood, energy, sleep, and anxiety levels. Your own experience, supported by the tools described in this chapter, will reveal what works best for your unique physiology. This is the foundation of sustainable, lifelong metabolic and emotional health.

References

Hall, H., Perelman, D., Breschi, A., Limcaoco, P., Kellogg, R., McLaughlin, T., & Snyder, M. P. (2018). Glucotypes reveal new patterns of glucose dysregulation. *PLOS Biology,* 16(7), e2005143. https://doi.org/10.1371/journal.pbio.2005143

Zeevi, D., Korem, T., Zmora, N., Israeli, D., Rothschild, D., Weinberger, A., … & Segal, E. (2015). Personalised nutrition by prediction of glycaemic responses. *Cell*, 163(5), 1079–1094. https://doi.org/10.1016/j.cell.2015.11.001

Danne, T., Nimri, R., Battelino, T., Bergenstal, R. M., Close, K. L., DeVries, J. H., … & Phillip, M. (2017). International consensus on use of continuous glucose monitoring. *Diabetes Care,* 40(12), 1631–1640. https://doi.org/10.2337/dc17-1600

Segal, E., Tashjian, S. K., Gurbatri, C. R., Darst, R. P., Alm, E., Sonnenburg, E. D., … & Snyder, M. P. (2022). Personalized micronutrition to improve human health. *Nature Medicine,* 28(10), 2062–2071. https://doi.org/10.1038/s41591-022-02013-x

Evert, A. B., Dennison, M., Gardner, C. D., Gerstel, P. M., Lau, K. H. K., Metcalf, P. A., … & Wylie-Rosett, J. (2019). Nutrition practice guideline for type 1 and type 2 diabetes in adults: Individualising carbohydrate distribution. *Diabetes Care*, 42(5), 731–754. https://doi.org/10.2337/dci19-0028

Cui, X., Abduljalil, A., Manor, B. D., Peng, C. K., & Novak, V. (2014). Multi-scale glycaemic variability: A link to gray matter atrophy and cognitive decline in type 2 diabetes. *PLOS ONE,* 9(1), e86284. https://doi.org/10.1371/journal.pone.0086284

Chapter 19: Managing Real-Life Challenges and Life Stages

Metabolic Transformation Across the Lifespan

Introduction: Adapting strategies as biology changes

Blood sugar regulation does not stay the same across a lifetime. Hormonal transitions, ageing, stress, illness, and major life changes all shift the metabolic landscape in ways that require your approach to adapt. Rather than following a rigid protocol indefinitely, the goal is understanding how your biology changes at different life stages, so you can adjust your strategies as you move through them.

Pregnancy: Insulin Resistance, Gestational Diabetes, and Maternal Mental Health

Pregnancy creates a state of profound metabolic transformation. To ensure adequate glucose reaches the developing foetus, the placenta secretes **human placental lactogen (HPL)** and increases **progesterone**, both hormones that actively reduce maternal insulin sensitivity. This metabolic change is physiologically necessary and universal: insulin resistance naturally develops in the third trimester of every pregnancy, even in women without prior metabolic dysfunction. Fasting insulin levels nearly double; glucose tolerance declines; some degree of hyperglycaemia becomes the new normal.

For most pregnant women, this glucose dysregulation remains subclinical and resolves postpartum. However, approximately 10–15 per cent of pregnancies develop **gestational diabetes mellitus (GDM)**, glucose levels persistently exceeding diagnostic thresholds despite compensatory hyperinsulinaemia.

GDM is more common, particularly in older maternal age, obesity, and those with family history of type 2 diabetes.

The mental health implications of GDM are profound and often overlooked. Pregnant women with gestational diabetes have 2–3 times the risk of prenatal and postpartum depression and anxiety compared to euglycaemic pregnancies, independent of baseline psychiatric history. The mechanism is multifactorial: hyperglycaemia itself directly impairs mood-regulating neurotransmitter synthesis and increases neuroinflammation; untreated GDM increases inflammatory markers like CRP; the metabolic stress of severe dysglycaemia activates sympathetic nervous system tone and increases cortisol; maternal psychological stress about foetal health intensifies; some women experience reactive hypoglycaemia during treatment, triggering panic and anxiety.

Evidence-based dietary strategies for pregnancy differ from non-pregnant individuals: energy requirements increase (approximately 300 additional calories daily in second and third trimesters), protein requirements increase substantially, and "eating for two" must not justify consuming refined carbohydrates or excessive calories. Emphasis should be placed on:

- **Protein at each meal**: 25–30 g per meal (total daily approximately 70–100 g)
- **Abundant non-starchy vegetables**: at every meal, providing fibre, micronutrients, and minimal glucose impact
- **Whole grains when included**: steel-cut oats, brown rice, and other whole forms with added protein and fat to blunt glycaemic response
- **Quality fats**: avocado, olive oil, nuts, and mercury-conscious seafood choices like wild-caught salmon
- **Limited added sugars and refined carbohydrates**: particularly important in third trimester when insulin resistance peaks
- **Regular movement**: even light activity such as walking, swimming, or prenatal yoga improves glucose tolerance and mental health

For women diagnosed with gestational diabetes, dietary intervention is typically first-line; if diet alone does not achieve glucose targets, metformin (with an excellent safety profile in pregnancy) or insulin is added. The combination of appropriate diet, movement, monitoring, and medical management when needed produces excellent outcomes for both maternal and foetal health.

Post-Partum: Blood Sugar Crashes, Thyroid Disruption, and Mood Disorders

The postpartum period, particularly the first 3–6 months, is a high-risk window for mood disorders. Approximately 15–20 per cent of new mothers experience clinically significant postpartum depression; 10–15 per cent experience postpartum anxiety. While psychological and social factors such as sleep deprivation and stress are undoubtedly important, the metabolic underpinnings are equally significant and frequently overlooked.

Several metabolic changes happen simultaneously in the postpartum period. **First, rapid oestrogen decline** occurs within hours to days after placental delivery. Oestrogen supports insulin sensitivity; its dramatic withdrawal precipitates a rebound in insulin resistance. Fasting glucose and insulin levels, which normalised during pregnancy, spike again postpartum. Additionally, oestrogen is a cofactor for serotonin synthesis and function; its withdrawal directly impairs serotonergic tone independent of dietary factors.

Second, many postpartum women experience reactive hypoglycaemia, particularly if breastfeeding (which creates ongoing glucose demand to produce milk). Dramatic overnight glucose crashes with night sweats, anxiety, and palpitations are common but frequently misattributed to nocturnal panic attacks rather than glucose dysregulation. Continuous glucose monitoring often reveals profound nocturnal hypoglycaemia (drops to 2.8–3.5 mmol/L) that responds perfectly to increased evening carbohydrate intake or shorter fasting intervals.

Third, postpartum thyroid dysfunction is common, particularly in women with thyroid autoimmunity. Postpartum thyroiditis, immune-mediated inflammation of the thyroid, causes temporary hypothyroidism in up to 10 per cent of women, producing fatigue, depression, cognitive fog, and weight gain that is deeply demoralising when combined with sleep deprivation.

Metabolic strategies for postpartum mental health include:

- **Frequent, protein-rich meals and snacks**: 4–5 eating occasions daily to prevent nocturnal hypoglycaemia and stabilise glucose throughout the day
- **Particular attention to breakfast and evening meals**: skipped or low-protein breakfast sets up afternoon crashes and afternoon anxiety; inadequate evening carbohydrates predispose to nocturnal hypoglycaemia
- **Iron and B12 supplementation** if pregnancy depleted stores (pregnancy-related anaemia is common and exacerbates mood disturbance)
- **Vitamin D supplementation**: deficiency is epidemic postpartum and correlates with depression
- **Thyroid testing**: TSH, free T4, free T3, and TPO antibodies should be checked at 6 weeks postpartum if mood symptoms emerge
- **Adequate sleep support**: partnered support for night feeds to protect maternal sleep, which is metabolically and psychiatrically essential

Perimenopause and Menopause: Oestrogen's Central Role in Metabolic Health

The perimenopause, the 5–10 years preceding the final menstrual period, is characterised by erratic oestrogen production as ovarian function declines. Oestrogen is not merely a reproductive hormone; it is a central regulator of **metabolic health and neurobiological stability**. The loss of oestrogen's metabolic actions creates significant challenges for many women.

Oestrogen enhances insulin secretion and insulin sensitivity at tissue level. As oestrogen declines, insulin resistance paradoxically worsens, not because behaviour has changed, but because the hormone supporting metabolic health is disappearing. Women often report that metabolic changes suddenly "flip" in perimenopause: a dietary approach that maintained stability for years abruptly fails to control blood sugar; previously stable weight begins creeping upward despite unchanged eating; new-onset anxiety or depressive episodes emerge.

Additionally, oestrogen supports **serotonin receptor expression** and serotonin transporter function; its decline directly impairs serotonergic neurotransmission. The combination of worsening insulin resistance, declining serotonin tone, and sleep disruption from hot flushes creates a "perfect storm" for depression and anxiety in midlife women.

Metabolic strategies for perimenopause and menopause are best viewed as proactive recalibration:

- **Reassess macronutrient distribution**: many women who thrived on moderate carbohydrate in youth find lower-carbohydrate approaches necessary in perimenopause to achieve equivalent glucose stability. This is not dietary failure; it is metabolic adaptation
- **Increase protein intake**: elevated protein (1.2–1.6 g per kg body weight) supports satiety, thermogenesis, and muscle preservation (sarcopenia accelerates with declining oestrogen)
- **Prioritise strength training**: resistance exercise is amongst the most effective interventions for preserving insulin sensitivity and muscle mass during the menopausal transition
- **Extend fasting windows cautiously**: many perimenopause women feel worse with extended fasting, perhaps because declining oestrogen increases cortisol sensitivity to fasting. Listen to your body
- **Consider hormone replacement therapy (HRT) if appropriate**: well-managed HRT can restore oestrogen's metabolic benefits and deeply improve mood, alongside dietary optimisation

Older Adulthood: Sarcopenia, Declining Insulin Sensitivity, and Cognitive Risk

Ageing is accompanied by progressive loss of muscle mass (**sarcopenia**), declining physical activity, and worsening insulin sensitivity, a trajectory almost guaranteed without active intervention. Simultaneously, cognitive decline accelerates; dementia risk rises exponentially after age 65; depression and anxiety become increasingly prevalent.

The metabolic contributions to cognitive decline are substantial. Insulin resistance itself is now understood as a core driver of Alzheimer's dementia, with some researchers referring to dementia as "type 3 diabetes." Hyperglycaemia impairs cerebral glucose utilisation, causes neuroinflammation, and accelerates accumulation of amyloid-beta and tau. Individuals with well-controlled glucose metabolism have significantly lower dementia risk than those with dysglycaemia.

Metabolic strategies for cognitive health in older adulthood include:

- **Aggressive preservation of muscle mass**: resistance training 2–3 times weekly is essential for maintaining insulin sensitivity and supporting glucose clearance
- **Protein intake at upper end of recommendations**: 1.2–1.5 g per kg body weight, distributed across meals to optimise muscle protein synthesis
- **Frequent movement throughout the day**: even short walks before and after meals significantly blunt postprandial glucose spikes
- **Sleep prioritisation**: cognitive decline accelerates with poor sleep; protection of sleep becomes essential
- **Cognitive training and learning**: novel learning activates glucose utilisation in the brain and may provide reserve against decline
- **Social engagement**: isolation is an independent risk factor for cognitive decline; strong social connections are amongst the most potent longevity factors

Social Eating, Restaurants, and Perfectionism-Free Strategies

A common concern is: "If I implement these dietary changes, will I be able to eat normally at restaurants and social gatherings?" The answer is yes, and rigid perfectionism is itself counterproductive to both metabolic health and mental wellbeing.

The problem with perfectionism is bidirectional: rigid avoidance of "forbidden" foods often leads to reactive overeating when willpower inevitably lapses; viewing occasional deviation from optimal diet as "failure" creates shame and anxiety that paradoxically worsen mood and trigger stress-eating.

Sustainable approaches to social eating include:

- **Eat normally and enjoyably**: your baseline diet matters far more than occasional social meals. One pizza dinner does not undo weeks of stable eating

- **Make intentional choices**: rather than mindlessly consuming what is served, decide what appeals to you and what aligns with your metabolic needs
- **Maintain protein and fibre**: even in social eating contexts, prioritising protein and vegetable sides blunts glycaemic impact
- **Alcohol strategy**: alcohol impairs liver glucose output, precipitating reactive hypoglycaemia hours later, particularly if consumed with minimal food. If drinking, eat substantial food simultaneously and monitor mood and sleep the following days
- **Plan ahead for predictable events**: if attending a wedding or buffet, decide in advance what foods appeal and what your approach will be
- **Forgive imperfection**: intermittent indulgences are compatible with metabolic health. What matters is the overall trajectory, not perfection on any single day

Shift Work and Circadian Metabolic Disruption

Shift workers, particularly those working overnight or rotating shifts, face a unique metabolic challenge: their eating patterns are reversed relative to circadian rhythms evolved for eating during daylight and sleeping at night. The metabolic consequences are substantial.

Circadian desynchrony (misalignment between behavioural schedules and endogenous circadian rhythms) impairs glucose tolerance independent of diet or activity. Individuals working overnight shifts have higher fasting glucose, higher HbA1c, elevated triglycerides, and greater insulin resistance than matched individuals working daytime hours. Additionally, circadian desynchrony impairs sleep quality and worsens mood regulation.

Metabolic strategies for shift workers include:

- **Maintain meal consistency**: eating three meals at consistent times relative to sleep (not clock time) helps. If you sleep 7am–3pm, eat "breakfast" upon waking and "dinner" before sleeping, even though these are unconventional clock times

- **Light exposure strategy**: bright light exposure during work hours signals "daytime" to your circadian clock; complete darkness during sleep hours preserves sleep quality
- **Melatonin supplementation**: 0.5–3 mg melatonin taken 30 minutes before desired sleep time helps shift circadian rhythms and improves sleep quality
- **Minimise caffeine late in your "evening"**: avoid caffeine 6–8 hours before your desired sleep time, even if that is daytime
- **Accept metabolic compromise**: despite optimization efforts, circadian misalignment unavoidably impairs glucose metabolism. Working with a healthcare provider to monitor glucose more closely is important

Acute Stress Events and the Fight-or-Flight Glucose Surge

Beyond chronic stress, acute stressors, relationship conflict, professional crisis, bereavement, illness, trigger an immediate, dramatic physiological response: **sympathetic nervous system activation** and massive release of cortisol and adrenaline. Part of this response is a glucose spike independent of food intake. The liver dramatically increases glucose output; cells reduce glucose uptake; blood glucose can surge 3–5 mmol/L within minutes even without eating.

For many people with anxiety or trauma history, these glucose spikes themselves trigger panic: the rapid heartbeat, sweating, trembling, and sense of imminent catastrophe during acute stress activate similar symptoms to hypoglycaemia. Understanding that acute glucose surges are an expected, temporary, normalising physiological response to stress can reduce secondary anxiety. Over time, the glucose surge dissipates as the acute stressor resolves or you psychologically adapt to it.

Strategies during acute stress include:

- **Breathing practices**: slow, deliberate breathing (6 breaths per minute) activates parasympathetic tone and blunts catecholamine release
- **Movement**: physical activity during acute stress helps metabolise the glucose surge and adrenaline mobilisation

- **Hydration and electrolytes**: maintain fluid and electrolyte intake during prolonged stress
- **Social support**: reaching out to trusted others activates parasympathetic tone through the vagal brake, attenuating the physiological stress response
- **Cognitive reframing**: reminding yourself that the glucose spike is a temporary, normal response to stress reduces secondary anxiety

Building Metabolic Resilience Through Consistent Daily Anchors

Rather than viewing blood sugar management as a series of discrete, situational rules, the most sustainable approach involves building **metabolic resilience**, the capacity to maintain stability across variable environments and stressors. Resilience emerges not from perfection but from consistent, daily practices that become automatic even during chaos.

Daily anchors that build resilience include:

- **Consistent meal timing**: eating at approximately the same times daily allows your digestive system to anticipate and prepare
- **Movement after meals**: a 2–3 minute walk after lunch and dinner dramatically attenuates postprandial glucose spikes
- **Sleep protection**: consistent sleep and wake times preserve circadian stability and sleep quality
- **Stress-management practices**: a daily meditation, yoga, or breathwork practice prevents stress accumulation
- **Social connection**: regular contact with trusted others, whether daily conversation or weekly gatherings
- **Nature exposure**: brief daily outdoor time activates parasympathetic tone and improves mood independent of food choices

These practices, maintained consistently, create a metabolic and neurobiological foundation resilient to occasional dietary indulgence, stressful days, or travel disruption. It is the steady baseline that matters most.

Key Takeaways

- **Pregnancy naturally induces insulin resistance in the third trimester**; gestational diabetes elevates depression and anxiety risk, managed through dietary protein and fibre emphasis, movement, and monitoring
- **Postpartum period combines rapid oestrogen decline, reactive hypoglycaemia, and thyroid dysfunction**; frequent protein-rich meals, careful monitoring, and thyroid testing are essential
- **Perimenopause and menopause worsen insulin resistance and reduce serotonin tone**; macronutrient recalibration, strength training, and HRT consideration often necessary
- **Ageing requires aggressive muscle preservation through protein and resistance training** to maintain insulin sensitivity and prevent cognitive decline
- **Social eating and occasional indulgences are compatible with metabolic health**; perfectionism is counterproductive
- **Shift workers experience circadian-desynchrony-induced metabolic impairment**; meal timing consistency, light exposure strategy, and closer monitoring help mitigate
- **Acute stress triggers physiological glucose surges independent of food**; understanding this as normal prevents secondary anxiety
- **Daily anchors**, consistent meal timing, post-meal movement, sleep protection, stress practices, social connection, nature exposure, build resilience across life stages

Next Steps

Understanding your life stage is essential because it determines which metabolic strategies will serve you best. Rather than comparing your approach to others, use these frameworks to assess where you are biologically, are you managing pregnancy, perimenopause, shift work, or ageing?, and adapt accordingly. In the next chapter, we move beyond life stages to explore how to prevent chronic disease through early biomarker detection and establishment of lifelong healthy patterns.

References

Metzger, B. E., Lowe, L. P., Dyer, A. R., Trimble, E. R., Chaovarindr, U., Coustan, D. R., … & HAPO Study Cooperative Research Group. (2008). Hyperglycemia and adverse pregnancy outcomes. *New England Journal of Medicine*, 358(19), 1991–2002. https://doi.org/10.1056/NEJMoa0707943

Davis, S. R., Lambrinoudaki, I., Lumsden, M., Mishra, G. D., Pal, L., Rees, M., … & Villaseca, P. (2015). Menopause. *Nature Reviews Disease Primers*, 1, 15004. https://doi.org/10.1038/nrdp.2015.4

Kessler, R. C., Petukhova, M., Sampson, N. A., Zaslavsky, A. M., & Wittchen, H. U. (2012). Twelve-month and lifetime prevalence and lifetime morbid risk of anxiety and mood disorders in the United States. *International Journal of Methods in Psychiatric Research*, 21(3), 169–184. https://doi.org/10.1002/mpr.1359

Baker, L. D., Frank, L. L., Foster-Schubert, K., Green, P. S., Wilkinson, C. W., McTiernan, A., … & Craft, S. (2010). Aerobic exercise improves cognition for older adults with glucose intolerance, a risk factor for Alzheimer's disease. *Journal of Alzheimer's Disease*, 22(2), 569–579. https://doi.org/10.3233/JAD-2010-100768

Chapter 20: Preventive Measures for Long-Term Health

Detecting Disease Before Symptoms Emerge

Introduction: Prevention as the foundation of health

The most effective approach to long-term mental and physical health is not treating problems after they arise, it is catching metabolic dysfunction before it becomes diagnosable. Blood sugar dysregulation, insulin resistance, and nutrient depletion typically develop over years before producing symptoms. Knowing which biomarkers to monitor and how to interpret them gives you the capacity to intervene early, and to maintain genuine vitality, not just the absence of illness.

Metabolic Syndrome: From Silent Dysregulation to Psychiatric Crisis

Metabolic syndrome is a cluster of physiological abnormalities that co-occur: elevated fasting glucose or HbA1c, elevated triglycerides, reduced HDL cholesterol, elevated blood pressure, and increased central adiposity (particularly visceral fat around organs). Metabolic syndrome is diagnosed when an individual meets 3 of 5 criteria; it affects approximately 25–30 per cent of adults in developed nations and as many as 40 per cent of those over 60 years old.

Metabolic syndrome is clinically significant for two good reasons. First, individuals with metabolic syndrome have substantially elevated cardiovascular disease risk, myocardial infarction, stroke, sudden cardiac death. Second, metabolic syndrome is a potent driver of psychiatric illness. Studies across multiple populations demonstrate that individuals with metabolic syndrome have 2–3 times higher risk of depression, anxiety, and cognitive decline compared to metabolically healthy individuals. The relationship is bidirectional: depression impairs metabolic health through stress-driven dysglycaemia and reduced physical activity; metabolic dysregulation impairs mood through insulin resistance, neuroinflammation, and impaired neurotransmitter synthesis.

Critically, metabolic syndrome develops silently, it is entirely possible to have insulin resistance, elevated triglycerides, declining HDL, and elevated blood pressure without feeling anything amiss. A person may feel subjectively well, remain at a "normal" BMI, and exercise regularly whilst honouring serious metabolic dysfunction. **Early biomarker detection, testing before symptoms emerge, is therefore essential**.

Early Biomarker Detection: What to Test and How Often

A comprehensive metabolic assessment should extend beyond the standard cholesterol panel typically measured at annual physical exams. Understanding the following tests provides early warning of dysregulation and allows intervention before disease crystallises:

Fasting glucose (normal <5.5 mmol/L; prediabetic range 5.5–6.9 mmol/L) is informative but represents only a snapshot. Many people with prediabetes have normal fasting glucose; this test alone misses them.

Fasting insulin (optimal <5 mIU/L; borderline 5–10 mIU/L; elevated/insulin resistant >10 mIU/L) is arguably the single most important early warning sign. Elevated fasting insulin in the presence of normal glucose indicates the pancreas is oversecreeting to maintain normal glucose, a sign of declining tissue insulin sensitivity. Fasting insulin rises years before glucose elevation, making it the earliest harbinger of metabolic deterioration.

HbA1c (normal <5.5 per cent; prediabetic range 5.5–6.4 per cent) reflects 3-month average glucose and is stable across days. HbA1c becomes progressively elevated as dysglycaemia worsens, but by the time HbA1c is elevated, glucose dysregulation has typically persisted for months.

HOMA-IR (Homeostatic Model Assessment for Insulin Resistance) is calculated from fasting glucose and fasting insulin: HOMA-IR = (fasting glucose in mmol/L × fasting insulin in mIU/L) / 22.5. HOMA-IR >1.8 suggests significant insulin resistance and is associated with depression and cardiovascular disease independent of glucose level.

Lipid profile including total cholesterol, LDL, HDL, and triglycerides captures cardiovascular risk; elevated triglycerides (>1.7 mmol/L) indicate ongoing dysglycaemia and reflect glucose dysregulation more accurately than fasting glucose itself.

C-Reactive Protein (CRP), a systemic inflammation marker, is elevated in depression, anxiety, and dementia. CRP >3.0 mg/L indicates significant inflammation. Glucose dysregulation is a potent driver of CRP elevation; dietary stabilisation typically reduces CRP substantially.

Homocysteine (elevated if >12 µmol/L) is an amino acid associated with depression, cognitive decline, and vascular disease. Homocysteine elevation reflects impaired methylation, often from B vitamin insufficiency. Glucose dysregulation impairs the methylation cycle, raising homocysteine.

Liver function tests, particularly GGT (gamma-glutamyl transferase) and ALT (alanine aminotransferase), reflect fatty liver disease, increasingly prevalent in dysglycaemia. Fatty liver impairs glucose metabolism and is associated with depression.

Vitamin D (optimal 40–80 ng/mL; deficiency <20 ng/mL) is critical for immune function, mood regulation, and calcium metabolism. Deficiency is endemic in depression and seasonal affective disorder.

Thyroid panel including TSH, free T3, and free T4 (plus TPO antibodies if autoimmunity is suspected) is essential because thyroid dysfunction causes depression, anxiety, and fatigue often misattributed to primary psychiatric illness.

Recommended testing frequency: comprehensive metabolic panel (glucose, insulin, lipids, CRP, liver function, kidney function) every 1–2 years for metabolically healthy individuals; more frequently (6–12 monthly) if biomarkers are abnormal or risk factors are present. Annual vitamin D and thyroid testing is reasonable for those with psychiatric history or metabolic risk factors.

Fasting Insulin: The Earliest Warning Sign of Insulin Resistance

Fasting insulin deserves particular emphasis as the single most sensitive early indicator of metabolic deterioration. Understanding why requires brief biochemistry.

Insulin is a hormone secreted by pancreatic beta cells in response to elevated glucose. After a meal, glucose rises; insulin rises to facilitate glucose entry into cells. In metabolically healthy individuals, fasting insulin is low (3–5 mIU/L) because tissue insulin sensitivity is high, cells respond efficiently to insulin, so the pancreas need not oversecrete to maintain normal fasting glucose.

In insulin-resistant individuals, tissues respond sluggishly to insulin. The pancreas compensates by secreting more and more insulin to achieve the same glucose-lowering effect. Thus fasting insulin rises, sometimes to 15, 20, 30 mIU/L or higher, whilst glucose remains normal. This is **compensated insulin resistance**: the system is still maintaining glucose within normal range, but at cost of excessive insulin, which itself causes inflammation and contributes to psychiatric illness.

Over years to decades, this compensatory mechanism fails: the pancreas becomes exhausted or beta cells begin dying; glucose starts rising; prediabetes and eventually diabetes develop. But for years prior, fasting insulin has been silently rising, signalling the deterioration.

Importantly, fasting insulin is modifiable through lifestyle: a 3–6 month period of diet emphasising whole foods, fibre, protein, and healthy fats, combined with regular movement and sleep improvement, typically reduces elevated fasting insulin substantially, often dramatically. This early intervention interrupts the trajectory toward diabetes and its psychiatric sequelae.

Longevity Pathways: mTOR, Sirtuins, NAD+, and Their Dietary Triggers

An emerging paradigm in ageing science focuses on **longevity pathways**, cellular signalling cascades that regulate the pace of ageing. Understanding these pathways reveals how diet and lifestyle influence not just disease prevention but the rate of biological ageing itself.

mTOR (mechanistic target of rapamycin) is a nutrient sensor that detects abundant amino acids, glucose, and energy status. When mTOR is highly activated (which occurs with high protein/carbohydrate intake and excess calorie consumption), cells enter an anabolic, growth-promoting state: protein synthesis increases, cell division increases, energy is directed toward growth and reproduction. This state is protective early in life but, when sustained chronically, accelerates cellular senescence and ageing.

Conversely, **mTOR inhibition**, achieved through calorie restriction, fasting, and certain phytonutrients, shifts cells toward catabolic processes: autophagy (cellular "clean-up"), mitochondrial renewal, DNA repair, and stress-resistance pathways activate. Extended periods of mTOR inhibition appear to extend lifespan across organisms from yeast to primates.

Sirtuins (particularly SIRT1, SIRT3, SIRT6) are NAD+-dependent enzymes that activate longevity programmes. Sirtuins promote mitochondrial function, DNA repair, and metabolic flexibility. Sirtuin activation occurs during fasting, calorie restriction, and with specific dietary compounds like resveratrol (in red wine and berries) and quercetin (in apples and onions).

NAD+ (nicotinamide adenine dinucleotide) is a coenzyme critical for energy metabolism and sirtuins' function. NAD+ levels decline with ageing; supplementation via precursors like NMN or NR enhances mitochondrial function and appears to slow some aspects of ageing. Conversely, poor blood sugar control impairs NAD+ metabolism, and dysglycaemic individuals have lower NAD+ than metabolically healthy counterparts.

The practical implication: **periodic fasting or calorie restriction activates longevity pathways**, particularly if combined with high-intensity interval exercise. These are not merely weight-loss strategies but tools for altering the pace of ageing itself. Individuals who incorporate regular fasting often report improved metabolic biomarkers alongside subjective improvements in energy, clarity, and mood, possibly through activation of these rejuvenating cellular programmes.

Intermittent Fasting Protocols for Metabolic Health

Intermittent fasting, eating within a compressed time window, leaving 12–20+ hours without food, has emerged as a powerful metabolic intervention supported by substantial research. Multiple protocols exist.

16:8 (time-restricted eating) involves consuming all daily food within an 8-hour window (e.g., noon–8pm), fasting for 16 hours overnight and morning. This is the most sustainable for most people, it simply compresses normal eating into a shorter window without requiring calorie counting.

5:2 involves eating normally five days weekly; on two non-consecutive days, consuming only 500–600 calories (approximately 25 per cent of normal intake). This preserves the ability to eat normally on 5 days.

Eat-stop-eat involves extended 24-hour fasts once or twice weekly (e.g., finishing dinner at 7pm Monday, not eating until 7pm Tuesday, eating normally Wednesday).

Alternate-day fasting alternates between fast days (very low calorie or no food) and normal eating days.

Research in fasting demonstrates multiple benefits beyond weight loss: improved insulin sensitivity (fasting periods without food reduce insulin demand; during extended fasting, liver glycogen depletes and cells shift toward fat oxidation, reducing circulating insulin and improving tissue sensitivity); **autophagy activation** (extended fasting >16–18 hours activates autophagy, the cellular recycling process that clears damaged mitochondria, misfolded proteins, and senescent cells, a key longevity mechanism); improved mood and cognitive function (many individuals report improved mental clarity, reduced anxiety, and improved mood with regular fasting, possibly through ketone production and activation of longevity pathways); metabolic flexibility (regular fasting restores the body's ability to shift between glucose and fat oxidation).

Cautions with fasting: some individuals, particularly those with anxiety, trauma history, or eating disorder vulnerability, experience increased anxiety or disordered eating patterns with fasting. Individuals on psychiatric medications or with active mood disturbance should implement fasting cautiously and with professional guidance. Additionally, fasting is not appropriate during acute stress, illness, or recovery from illness; these states require adequate nutrition.

Polyphenols and Antioxidant-Rich Foods as Metabolic Protectors

Polyphenols are a class of plant compounds with powerful antioxidant and anti-inflammatory properties. They are found in abundance in colourful vegetables, berries, tea, coffee, dark chocolate, and olive oil. Research demonstrates that high polyphenol intake is associated with reduced insulin resistance, improved glucose control, lower CRP, and reduced dementia and depression risk.

Mechanisms include: reduced glucose absorption (some polyphenols slow carbohydrate absorption, blunting postprandial glucose spikes); improved insulin secretion (certain polyphenols enhance beta cell function and insulin release); antioxidant and anti-inflammatory effects (polyphenols reduce systemic inflammation and oxidative stress, protective against both metabolic disease and psychiatric illness); prebiotic effects (polyphenols feed beneficial gut bacteria, supporting healthy microbiota that improves metabolic health).

Practical polyphenol sources to emphasise include: coloured berries (blueberries, blackberries, cranberries), dark leafy greens (spinach, kale), colourful vegetables (purple cabbage, orange sweet potato, red bell pepper), green and white tea, coffee, extra-virgin olive oil, dark chocolate (≥70 per cent cacao), nuts (walnuts, almonds), and herbs (turmeric, oregano, thyme). A simple approach: "eating the rainbow", consuming vegetables and fruits across the spectrum of colours, ensures diverse polyphenol intake.

Social Connection as an Independent Longevity Variable

Decades of longitudinal research demonstrate that **social connection is amongst the most potent determinants of health and longevity**, rivalling smoking, alcohol, obesity, physical activity, and diet in impact. Individuals with strong social relationships have 50 per cent lower mortality risk than isolated individuals; the effect is independent of any medical intervention.

The mechanisms linking social connection to longevity are complex. Social interaction activates the vagal brake, shifting from sympathetic fight-or-flight dominance to parasympathetic rest-and-digest tone, reducing cortisol, blood pressure, and inflammation whilst improving glucose regulation. Social isolation is a potent risk factor for both psychiatric illness and metabolic disease; strong relationships are protective. Individuals with strong social support are more likely to exercise, eat healthily, sleep well, and engage in stress-management practices. Positive social interaction upregulates immune function, improving infection resistance and potentially slowing cancer progression.

From a mental health perspective, social connection is not merely supportive during difficulties, it is foundational to mental health itself. Individuals without close relationships, regardless of diet or exercise, are at substantially elevated psychiatric risk. Conversely, individuals with strong social bonds experience better mental health even during metabolic dysregulation.

Practical implementation involves prioritising regular contact with people who matter: weekly phone calls or meals with friends or family, participation in group activities (sports, classes, volunteer organisations), cultivating a sense of community. Even brief, positive social interaction provides measurable health benefit.

The Compounding Effect: Why Small Daily Habits Matter More Than Occasional Interventions

A final principle: metabolic and mental health improvement follows a **compounding curve**, not a linear relationship. Small daily choices, a morning walk, eating protein with breakfast, drinking water before meals, an evening wind-down practice, seem negligible in isolation. Over one day they are trivial. Over one week, their impact remains modest. Over months and years, however, they create profound transformation.

This is why a person who walks 15 minutes daily will experience greater metabolic improvement over two years than someone who completes a single week-long intensive diet or exercise programme. Likewise, consistently stable blood sugar across 300 days creates far greater benefits than perfection for 30 days followed by return to baseline.

The inverse is equally true: small daily dysregulations compound. A person consuming slightly excessive simple carbohydrates daily, accumulating slightly impaired sleep nightly, experiencing chronic low-grade stress, these individuals show accelerated metabolic deterioration over years despite appearing relatively stable from day-to-day.

Understanding compounding should shift motivation from **pursuing dramatic transformations** ("I will do a 30-day cleanse, then return to normal") to **establishing sustainable daily practices** that persist indefinitely. The goal is not perfection but the consistent, boring repetition of behaviour aligned with health.

For those struggling with motivation, focusing on **habit stacking**, anchoring new practices to existing daily routines, makes sustainability easier. "After I pour my morning coffee, I will drink a glass of water." "After lunch, I will take a 5-minute walk." "Before bed, I will spend 10 minutes in breathwork." These tiny additions, accumulated, transform life.

Key Takeaways

- **Metabolic syndrome is silent and common**, affecting 25–40 per cent of adults, and is a potent driver of psychiatric illness; early detection through biomarker testing enables prevention
- **Fasting insulin is the earliest indicator of insulin resistance**, rising years before glucose elevation, making it the most sensitive test for metabolic intervention
- **Longevity pathways** (mTOR, sirtuins, NAD+) are activated through periodic fasting, calorie restriction, and high-polyphenol foods; activating these pathways may slow biological ageing
- **Intermittent fasting protocols** (16:8, 5:2) improve insulin sensitivity, activate autophagy, and improve mental clarity in many individuals; implement cautiously in those with mood instability or eating disorder vulnerability

- **High-polyphenol foods** (berries, leafy greens, coloured vegetables, tea, coffee) reduce insulin resistance and inflammation through multiple mechanisms
- **Social connection is amongst the most potent longevity and mental health factors**, rivalling diet and exercise in impact; prioritise regular meaningful relationships
- **Metabolic improvement compounds over time**; small daily consistent practices create far greater long-term benefit than occasional intensive interventions
- **Sustainable health emerges from boring daily habits**, not dramatic protocols; habit stacking makes adoption easier

Next Steps

You now understand how to test for metabolic dysfunction before it becomes disease, and how lifestyle practices that activate longevity pathways can extend healthy lifespan. The next challenge is understanding why these practices are becoming increasingly necessary, how the food supply itself has transformed over recent decades, creating metabolic vulnerability for millions. This understanding will deepen your commitment to metabolic stability.

References

El-Osta, A., Brasacchio, D., Yao, D., Xian, M., Froguel, P., Wolff, G., … & Brownlee, M. (2008). Transient high glucose causes persistent epigenetic changes and altered gene expression during subsequent normoglycemia. *Journal of Experimental Medicine*, 205(10), 2409–2417. https://doi.org/10.1084/jem.20081692

Biessels, G. J., Staekenborg, S., Brunner, E., Brayne, C., & Scheltens, P. (2006). Risk of dementia in diabetes mellitus: A systematic review. *The Lancet Neurology*, 5(1), 64–74. https://doi.org/10.1016/S1474-4422(05)70284-2

Pedersen, B. K., & Saltin, B. (2015). Exercise as medicine, evidence for prescribing exercise as therapy in 26 different chronic diseases. *Scandinavian Journal of Medicine & Science in Sports*, 25(S3), 1–72.

https://doi.org/10.1111/sms.12581

Baudrand, R., & Vaidya, A. (2015). The cortisol connection: Primary aldosteronism, glucocorticoids, and metabolic disease. *Current Opinion in Endocrinology, Diabetes and Obesity*, 22(3), 222–229. https://doi.org/10.1097/MED.0000000000000158
https://doi.org/10.1161/HYPERTENSIONAHA.115.05628

Chapter 21: How Food Has Changed – The Rise of Processed Foods and Addiction

The Engineered Food Supply and Your Brain

Introduction: Why metabolic vulnerability is increasing

If you have ever found it difficult to eat well despite knowing better, there is a reason, and it is not a lack of willpower. The modern food supply has been systematically engineered to override satiety signals, hijack reward circuitry, and drive overconsumption of exactly the foods that destabilise blood sugar. Understanding how this happened, and who benefits from it, reframes the struggle with food as a systemic problem rather than a personal failure.

The Transformation of the Food Supply

In recent decades, processed foods have become a major part of the average diet, transforming the way we eat and our relationship with food. Unlike whole foods, processed foods are often engineered to be hyper-palatable, designed to trigger pleasure responses in the brain, making them more addictive and driving over-consumption.

Dr Robert Lustig, an expert on sugar and metabolic health, has documented how the food industry has systematically altered products to maximise palatability and consumption by adjusting the precise ratio of sugar, fat, and salt to produce a "bliss point", a combination that the brain's reward centres find uniquely compelling. Dr David Kessler, former FDA Commissioner, has described this cycle as "conditioned hyper-eating," where people find themselves eating more than they intend, driven by intense cravings that are not easily overcome by willpower alone.

Processed foods are engineered to be quickly absorbed and low in fibre, leading to rapid blood sugar spikes and crashes. These fluctuations cause cravings, irritability, and fatigue, creating a cycle that encourages further consumption of sugary or high-fat foods to regain energy. The cravings and loss of control are not personal weakness, they are rational responses to dysglycaemia created by the food itself.

The Commercial Forces Shaping Dietary Behaviour

The impact of the food industry extends beyond individual health to shape dietary norms and food availability worldwide. Processed foods are cheap to produce, have a long shelf life, and are convenient, making them widely accessible. As a result, they have become staples in many households, contributing to the rise in obesity, diabetes, depression, and other chronic conditions.

Understanding the commercial and structural forces driving food choices is important for building genuine resilience against them. Marketing, food environment design, school canteens, workplace cafeterias, and the relative cost of whole versus processed foods all influence dietary behaviour in ways that individual willpower alone cannot overcome. This is not a failure of personal discipline, it is a rational response to an environment deliberately engineered to encourage over-consumption.

Advocacy for food policy change, including sugar taxes, restrictions on marketing to children, and improved labelling, complements individual dietary changes. By recognising these systemic forces, you can work to influence them whilst simultaneously making choices within your current environment.

Reclaiming Your Plate: Practical Strategies for Dietary Change

Practical strategies for reducing processed food dependence include:

- **Shop the perimeter of the store**: Fresh produce, meats, dairy, and other whole foods are typically located on the outer edges of supermarkets, whilst processed and packaged foods occupy the centre aisles

- **Cook at home**: Preparing meals at home gives direct control over ingredients, allowing the use of fresh, whole foods and avoiding added sugars, unhealthy fats, and preservatives
- **Plan ahead**: Meal planning and batch cooking reduce reliance on convenience foods during busy periods
- **Limit sugary drinks**: Replace sodas, sweetened teas, and juice drinks with water, herbal teas, or sparkling water
- **Acknowledge the addictive design**: Recognising that processed foods are engineered to override normal satiety signals can reduce self-blame and support more compassionate, effective behaviour change

By shifting perspective from "I am weak" to "I am responding rationally to a deliberately manipulative food environment," you access self-compassion and clarity that make dietary change sustainable.

The Global Malnutrition Paradox: Overfed and Undernourished

One of the most striking paradoxes of modern global health is the simultaneous occurrence of childhood obesity and childhood stunting, stunting referring to abnormally low height for age, a marker of chronic malnutrition, often in the same countries and sometimes in the same communities. Recent data documents that whilst 188 million children globally are overweight or obese, 149 million are stunted. In many low- and middle-income countries, these two forms of malnutrition coexist, creating populations that are simultaneously overfed and undernourished.

This paradox reflects a fundamental truth about ultra-processed foods: they provide abundant calories whilst remaining extraordinarily nutrient-poor. A diet consisting primarily of refined grains, sugary snacks, processed meats, and vegetable oil-based products delivers thousands of calories daily whilst providing negligible amounts of vitamins, minerals, fibre, and phytonutrients. An obese child eating predominantly ultra-processed foods may simultaneously be deficient in vitamin A, iron, zinc, and B vitamins, the same micronutrients essential for brain development, mood stability, and immune function.

The psychiatric cost of this nutritional paradox is staggering. **Obesity in women is associated with a 37 per cent increase in major depression.** Young females with obesity are **43 per cent more likely to develop anxiety disorders** compared to their lean peers. These are not minor epidemiological associations; they reflect the real human cost of metabolic dysfunction driven by nutritional bankruptcy.

Critically, refined sugars actively deplete intracellular stores of B vitamins (B1, B2, B3, B5, B6, B12), magnesium, zinc, and chromium, the precise cofactors required for insulin signal transduction, dopamine and serotonin synthesis, and cellular antioxidative defence. Ultra-processed food consumption creates a pathophysiological state of profound nutritional bankruptcy whilst simultaneously driving metabolic dysfunction. This state of simultaneous caloric excess and micronutrient depletion directly drives psychiatric vulnerability.

The Hidden Cost: How Nutrient Deficiency Manifests as Psychiatric Illness

The implications for mental health are profound. Many of the mental health symptoms emerging in children and adolescents, depression, anxiety, ADHD-like presentations, emotional dysregulation, may reflect not primarily psychiatric pathology but rather nutrient deficiency in the context of caloric excess. A child with adequate calories but insufficient micronutrients for neurotransmitter synthesis, mitochondrial function, and antioxidant defence may present with classic depression symptoms, low mood, reduced motivation, poor concentration, when the underlying problem is remediable micronutrient insufficiency.

Developing nations face a particularly acute version of this problem: as traditional, micronutrient-rich whole foods are displaced by industrially produced ultra-processed imports, populations experience rapid rises in obesity and metabolic disease accompanied paradoxically by increasing rates of malnutrition-related illness and mental health problems. The epidemic of mental illness in teenagers and young adults in lower-income countries tracks closely with the expansion of ultra-processed food availability.

Depression and anxiety may not be purely psychological, they may reflect dysglycaemia and micronutrient insufficiency that dietary change can powerfully address.

Systems Change and Personal Agency

Addressing this paradox requires systemic change, prioritising whole, minimally processed foods, rebuilding food systems around nutrient density rather than caloric delivery, and ensuring that economic access to whole foods becomes more feasible than current reliance on cheap ultra-processed alternatives. At the individual level, it means understanding that weight management and mental health improvement are inseparable from micronutrient adequacy.

The good news is that dietary change is powerful. By prioritising whole foods, ensuring adequate protein and fibre, and attending to micronutrient status, you simultaneously improve metabolic health, glucose stability, and mental health. These changes are not competing goals, they are convergent. The very foods that stabilise your blood sugar also provide the micronutrients your brain needs for neurotransmitter synthesis and optimal mood regulation.

Key Takeaways

- **Modern processed foods are engineered to be hyper-palatable**, triggering reward pathways and driving over-consumption that individual willpower cannot easily resist
- **The food industry systematically manipulates sugar, fat, and salt ratios** to create a "bliss point" that maximises consumption; this is not personal weakness
- **Processed foods create rapid blood sugar spikes and crashes**, driving cravings, irritability, and fatigue that create a vicious cycle of over-consumption
- **The malnutrition paradox**: ultra-processed foods provide abundant calories whilst remaining nutrient-poor, creating populations that are simultaneously overfed and undernourished

- **Obesity is associated with a 37 per cent increase in depression**; young females with obesity are 43 per cent more likely to develop anxiety disorders
- **Refined sugars actively deplete B vitamins, magnesium, zinc, and chromium**, cofactors essential for mood stability and neurotransmitter synthesis
- **Many psychiatric symptoms in children and adolescents** may reflect nutrient deficiency in the context of caloric excess, remediable through dietary restoration
- **Systemic change is necessary** but complements individual dietary choices; shopping the perimeter, cooking at home, and planned meal preparation build resilience within your current environment

Next Steps

Now that you understand why the processed food environment makes metabolic stability challenging, the next step is to measure your individual glucose responses with precision. Continuous glucose monitoring provides unprecedented visibility into how your body actually responds to foods, stress, sleep, and activity, information that enables targeted, personalised intervention far more effective than generic dietary guidelines. This is the shift from understanding the problem to solving it.

References

Lustig, R. H. (2013). *Fat chance: Beating the odds against sugar, processed food, obesity, and disease.* Hudson Street Press.

Kessler, D. A. (2009). *The end of overeating: Taking control of the insatiable American appetite.* Rodale Books.

Moss, M. (2013). *Salt sugar fat: How the food giants hooked us.* Random House.

Gearhardt, A. N., Corbin, W. R., & Brownell, K. D. (2009). Food addiction: An examination of the diagnostic criteria for dependence. *Journal of Addiction*

Medicine, 3(1), 1–7. https://doi.org/10.1097/ADM.0b013e318193c993

Monteiro, C. A., Cannon, G., Levy, R. B., Moubarac, J. C., Louzada, M. L. C., Rauber, F., … & Jaime, P. C. (2019). Ultra-processed foods: What they are and how to identify them. *Public Health Nutrition*, 22(5), 936–941. https://doi.org/10.1017/S1368980018003762

Chapter 22: Continuous Glucose Monitoring – Real-Time Insights for Mental Wellness

Measuring What Matters Most

Introduction: From blind spots to precise data

For the first time in history, it is possible to measure your blood glucose non-invasively, continuously, and every few minutes around the clock. Continuous glucose monitoring (CGM), a technology originally developed for insulin-dependent diabetes, is now accessible to anyone, without a prescription. For those investigating the connection between blood sugar and mental health, it is transformative: instead of guessing which foods affect your mood, you can see it in real time.

How CGM Sensors Work: The Technology Behind the Data

A CGM is a small electrochemical sensor approximately the size of a postage stamp, worn on the skin, typically the back of the upper arm, abdomen, or thigh, that measures glucose concentration in **interstitial fluid** (the fluid surrounding cells) every 5–15 minutes. Electrochemical sensors work by a glucose oxidase reaction: glucose in the interstitial fluid reacts with an enzyme on the sensor, creating an electrical signal proportional to glucose concentration. This signal is amplified by a transmitter and transmitted wirelessly to a smartphone app or separate receiver, providing real-time glucose readings and trend arrows.

The distinction between **plasma glucose** (measured by finger-prick blood tests) and **interstitial glucose** (measured by CGMs) is important. Plasma glucose is the gold standard laboratory measurement; interstitial glucose lags plasma glucose by approximately 5 minutes and is approximately 8–10 per cent lower. For practical purposes, CGM readings are acceptably accurate for identifying patterns, though they are not precise enough to replace blood tests for clinical diagnosis of diabetes.

Common CGM systems include:

- **Abbott FreeStyle Libre**: applied to back of arm, worn for 14 days, requires scanning (no automatic transmission), relatively inexpensive, available in Australia without prescription
- **Dexcom G6/G7**: applied to abdomen, worn for 10–14 days, continuous automatic transmission to smartphone, higher cost, requires prescription in some regions
- **Medtronic Guardian**: integrated with insulin pump systems, continuous transmission, primarily for insulin-dependent diabetes
- **Eversense**: implanted subcutaneously for up to 90 days, niche application, rarely used outside clinical research

For individuals interested in exploring CGM for mental health and metabolic wellness optimisation, FreeStyle Libre and Dexcom G6/G7 are most practical and accessible.

What CGM Reveals That HbA1c and Fasting Glucose Miss: Glycaemic Variability

A fundamental limitation of traditional blood glucose testing is that **it captures only static snapshots**: a fasting glucose test shows glucose at one moment after 8 hours of fasting; an HbA1c shows average glucose over 3 months. These tests completely miss the intra-day variability, the glucose spikes, crashes, and turbulence, that occurs throughout every day.

Research using CGMs in non-diabetic, apparently metabolically healthy populations has revealed a striking finding: approximately 80 per cent of people classified as "metabolically healthy" by conventional tests (normal fasting glucose, normal HbA1c) experience significant post-meal glucose excursions, reactive hypoglycaemia, and day-to-day variability that conventional testing entirely misses. This "hidden glucose variability" is now understood to be a potent driver of inflammation, impaired mood, and cognitive dysfunction independent of absolute glucose levels.

For example, a person might have perfectly normal fasting glucose (4.8 mmol/L) and normal HbA1c (5.2 per cent), yet eat a high-carbohydrate breakfast and experience a glucose spike to 8.5 mmol/L, followed by a crash to 3.6 mmol/L (mild hypoglycaemia) at mid-morning. This entire pattern is invisible to traditional testing but deeply visible on CGM and directly correlates with mood instability, anxiety, and impaired concentration that the person experiences throughout the morning.

Research on CGM in Healthy and Non-Diabetic Populations

Over the past several years, scientific literature on CGM use in non-diabetic populations has expanded substantially, revealing compelling correlations between glucose patterns and mental health outcomes.

A landmark 2023 study published in *Nutrients* examined glucose patterns in healthy individuals using CGMs and found that **high glucose variability** (measured by coefficient of variation, with normal <20 per cent) was associated with poorer mood, increased irritability, and lower cognitive performance scores, even in the absence of diabetes. Individuals with variability >25 per cent reported significantly higher anxiety scores and lower mental wellbeing.

A 2024 Stanford University study using CGMs in healthy older adults found that **mean daily glucose variability was significantly associated with poorer performance on executive function, memory, and processing speed tests**, independent of diabetes diagnosis. The association was particularly pronounced in those with high variability, suggesting that variability, not absolute glucose level, is the key driver of cognitive impairment.

A 2023 study in the *Journal of Psychiatric Research* enrolled individuals with major depressive disorder and found that those with CGM-documented glucose variability greater than age-matched non-depressed controls showed more severe depressive symptoms. Importantly, dietary interventions that reduced glucose variability (lowering refined carbohydrates, adding protein and fat to meals) produced measurable improvements in depression severity scores over 12 weeks, independent of weight loss.

Additionally, research from the Levels Health initiative (a consumer CGM data platform aggregating data from thousands of users) documented that **post-meal glucose peak magnitude** correlates with subsequent mood and energy crashes: individuals whose glucose rises more than 2.2 mmol/L above fasting level after meals experience significantly more frequent afternoon energy crashes, irritability, and impaired focus than those with smaller peaks.

Glucose Patterns and Their Correlation with Mood, Anxiety, and Cognitive Performance

CGM studies have identified several glucose patterns correlating with specific mental health presentations.

Pattern 1: High postprandial peaks (glucose spikes >2.2 mmol/L above baseline within 60–90 minutes of eating) correlate with afternoon energy crashes, afternoon anxiety, and difficulty concentrating mid-to-late afternoon. The mechanism is bidirectional: the high glucose spike triggers excessive insulin release; as glucose falls rapidly, reactive counter-regulatory hormone release (cortisol and adrenaline) occurs, creating anxiety-like symptoms (rapid heart rate, trembling, sense of dread). Many individuals with afternoon anxiety attributed entirely to psychological causes find relief by preventing morning and midday glucose spikes.

Pattern 2: Reactive hypoglycaemia (glucose drops below 3.9 mmol/L in hours following meals) is particularly common in individuals with anxiety and panic disorder. The symptoms of hypoglycaemia (rapid heart rate, trembling, sweating, sense of impending catastrophe, difficulty thinking clearly) are nearly identical to panic attack symptoms. CGM often reveals that recurrent "panic attacks" are actually hypoglycaemic episodes triggered by prior meals. Addressing the preceding meal (adding protein and fat, reducing simple carbohydrates) resolves the anxiety entirely, a finding deeply reassuring to individuals who feared their anxiety was entirely psychological.

Pattern 3: Nocturnal hypoglycaemia (glucose dropping below 3.9 mmol/L during sleep) is common and often undetected without CGM. Individuals experience nocturnal awakening with pounding heart, sweating, nightmares, or sleep fragmentation. They and their clinicians often attribute these to anxiety or trauma-related sleep disturbance when CGM reveals a metabolic cause. Interventions addressing the preceding evening meal (delayed carbohydrates, increased fat and protein) often resolve nocturnal symptoms.

Pattern 4: High overall glucose variability (>25 per cent) with multiple spikes and crashes throughout the day correlates with emotional dysregulation, irritability, and bipolar-like mood oscillations. Individuals describe being "fine one moment, angry the next" without apparent trigger. Stabilising glucose through consistent protein intake, balanced macronutrients, and regular movement often produces dramatic improvements in emotional stability and reduction in angry outbursts.

Pattern 5: Consistently elevated glucose (>7 mmol/L for substantial periods) correlates with depression, cognitive fog, and poor motivation. The mechanisms include: reduced neurotrophic factor (BDNF) production, impaired serotonin synthesis, neuroinflammation. Individuals often report that when glucose levels are brought down, mental fog clears and motivation and mood improve within days to weeks.

Identifying Trigger Foods and Personal Glycaemic Responses

Perhaps the most practical value of CGM is identifying foods that cause problematic glucose responses for you as an individual. Recall that identical foods produce vastly different responses in different people: a banana causes modest elevation in one person but dramatic spiking in another; oatmeal, widely promoted as healthy, produces large spikes in many individuals but minimal response in others.

CGM reveals your individual responses with precision. Over a 2-week wear period, you can systematically test foods, observe your individual response, and identify which foods are metabolically problematic for you specifically. For example:

- You might discover that your preferred breakfast (granola with yoghurt and fruit) produces a spike to 8.9 mmol/L, followed by a crash to 3.4

mmol/L at 10:30am, which correlates with mid-morning anxiety. Swapping the granola for nuts and maintaining the yoghurt and fruit eliminates the spike and anxiety

- You might find that you tolerate moderate amounts of whole-grain bread but react poorly to refined white bread, or that you tolerate fruit well earlier in the day but not after 4pm when insulin sensitivity naturally declines
- You might discover that adding a tablespoon of fat (olive oil, butter, nut butter) or protein (eggs, cheese) to a carbohydrate-containing meal you normally eat blunts the glucose spike substantially

This individualised learning is powerful because it is experiential, immediate, and self-directed. You observe your own data and make conclusions, far more motivating and sustainable than following generic dietary guidelines.

The Dawn Phenomenon and Its Mental Health Implications

Dawn phenomenon (also called "dawn effect") is the early-morning glucose rise that occurs in many people in the hours before waking. It occurs because cortisol and growth hormone, which naturally rise in the early morning to promote awakening and early-day activity, simultaneously increase hepatic glucose output. Glucose may rise 0.5–2.0 mmol/L or more between 3am and 7am without any food consumption.

For individuals with glucose dysregulation, dawn phenomenon can be pronounced, with fasting glucose potentially 1.5–2.0 mmol/L higher than evening glucose despite overnight fasting. This manifests as waking anxious, irritable, or foggy, symptoms many individuals attribute to poor sleep quality or anxiety but which CGM reveals to be glucose-related.

The mental health implications include: early-morning anxiety (waking with racing heart, sense of dread, or inability to calm thoughts is common with pronounced dawn phenomenon); morning irritability (waking mood instability that improves after breakfast correlates with dawn phenomenon); impaired morning clarity (cognitive fog upon waking, with improvement later in the day, reflects elevated early-morning glucose).

Strategies for managing dawn phenomenon include:

- **Evening carbohydrate consumption**: paradoxically, adding modest carbohydrates to the evening meal can reduce dawn phenomenon by providing hepatic glycogen and reducing the magnitude of overnight glucose output
- **Protein before bed**: a small protein-containing snack before sleep (Greek yoghurt, handful of nuts, cheese) blunts overnight hepatic glucose output
- **Evening movement**: a short walk after dinner improves overnight glucose stability
- **Sleep quality**: poor sleep exacerbates dawn phenomenon; prioritising sleep improves overnight glucose
- **Stress management**: evening stress raises cortisol, which worsens dawn phenomenon; evening meditation or breathwork helps

Glycaemic Variability Metrics: Standard Deviation, Time in Range, MAGE

CGM data are complex; interpreting it requires understanding key metrics.

Time in Range (TIR) is the percentage of time glucose remains within a target range. For non-diabetic individuals, target range is typically 3.9–7.8 mmol/L (70–140 mg/dL). Higher TIR correlates with better metabolic and mental health outcomes. TIR >90 per cent is considered excellent; TIR <70 per cent suggests significant dysregulation. Many individuals aim for TIR >85 per cent as a reasonable, sustainable target.

Glucose Variability (GV), measured by **Coefficient of Variation (CV)**, quantifies the degree of fluctuation throughout the day. CV = (standard deviation of glucose ÷ mean glucose) × 100. Normal CV <20 per cent; elevated CV >25–30 per cent indicates significant variability and is associated with mood instability and cognitive impairment. Some research suggests CV is more predictive of poor mental and cognitive outcomes than absolute glucose level.

Mean Amplitude of Glucose Excursions (MAGE) measures the average magnitude of glucose spikes and drops. MAGE <1.7 mmol/L is considered stable; MAGE >2.2 mmol/L indicates reactive dysglycaemia. High MAGE correlates with anxiety, irritability, and emotional dysregulation.

Post-Meal Peak (or postprandial peak) is the highest glucose reached within 2 hours of eating. For non-diabetics, post-meal peak is ideally <1.7–2.2 mmol/L above fasting glucose. Peaks >2.5 mmol/L above baseline indicate excessive insulin demand and increased risk of subsequent reactive hypoglycaemia.

Time Below Range (TBR), the percentage of time glucose drops below 3.9 mmol/L, is equally important to monitor. Even brief periods of hypoglycaemia trigger cortisol and adrenaline release, activating anxiety-like symptoms. TBR <5 per cent is reasonable; TBR >10 per cent suggests problematic reactive hypoglycaemia requiring dietary intervention.

How to Start: Sensor Placement, Calibration, and Reading the Data

Purchasing and wearing a CGM is straightforward. FreeStyle Libre is available in Australian pharmacies and online without prescription; cost is approximately $70–90 AUD per sensor (14-day wear). Dexcom systems are available through medical supply companies; cost is higher but may be covered partly by private health insurance depending on policy.

Sensor application involves: clean the application site (back of upper arm or abdomen) with soap and water; allow to dry; apply the adhesive pad firmly, ensuring good skin contact; insert the transmitter into the sensor; the system activates automatically. Most systems require 15–60 minutes of "warm-up" before accurate readings begin.

Initial calibration varies by system. FreeStyle Libre requires no calibration if sensor is inserted correctly. Dexcom systems typically require 2 finger-prick calibrations in the first day to ensure accuracy, then continue learning the individual's glucose patterns.

Reading and interpreting data is typically done via smartphone app. Key aspects to understand: **glucose value** (current glucose in mmol/L or mg/dL); **trend arrow** (arrow pointing up, level, or down indicates whether glucose is rising, stable, or falling and approximately how rapidly); **graph** (most apps display a continuous glucose trace for the past 3–24 hours, allowing you to see meal responses and glucose patterns); **notifications/alarms** (apps alert you if glucose rises above or falls below user-set thresholds; useful for catching spikes and hypoglycaemia).

Practical Protocol: A 2-Week CGM Experiment

A typical approach to deriving maximum insight from a 2-week CGM wear period involves systematic experimentation.

Week 1: Baseline observation. Wear the sensor without making deliberate changes; simply observe your natural glucose patterns. Document your meals, activity, sleep, stress, mood, and energy levels alongside glucose data. Identify patterns: Do spikes correlate with specific meals? Do crashes correlate with particular times or preceding meals? Do mood changes correspond to glucose changes?

Week 2: Targeted intervention. Based on Week 1 observations, implement targeted changes to meals or timing and observe the effect on glucose response. For example: if Week 1 revealed that breakfast causes spikes and crashes, try adding protein or fat to breakfast in Week 2 and observe if this stabilises glucose. If nocturnal hypoglycaemia was observed, add an evening carbohydrate or protein snack and assess the effect. Test one variable at a time to isolate cause and effect.

Documentation approach:

Create a simple spreadsheet with columns for:

- Date and time
- Meals eaten and approximate macronutrient composition (rough estimate: carb/protein/fat grams)
- Physical activity (type and duration)
- Sleep (duration and quality)
- Mood (0–10 scale)
- Energy level (0–10)

- Anxiety/irritability (0–10)
- Glucose metrics (if using an app with data export: peak glucose, time in range, variability)

Over 2 weeks, patterns emerge that link specific meals, timing, activity, or stress to glucose responses and mood changes.

Key Takeaways

- **CGM measures interstitial glucose continuously every 5–15 minutes**, revealing glucose patterns and variability that traditional fasting glucose and HbA1c testing completely miss
- **Approximately 80 per cent of metabolically healthy individuals experience hidden glucose variability** associated with mood instability, anxiety, and cognitive impairment despite normal conventional glucose tests
- **Post-meal glucose peaks, reactive hypoglycaemia, and high glucose variability correlate specifically with anxiety, irritability, mood crashes, and cognitive impairment**; identifying and addressing these patterns often resolves psychiatric symptoms
- **Individual food responses vary deeply**; CGM reveals your personal glycaemic response to specific foods, enabling personalised dietary optimisation far more effective than generic guidelines
- **Dawn phenomenon** (early-morning glucose rise from cortisol and growth hormone) contributes to morning anxiety and irritability in many individuals; evening carbohydrates, protein, and stress management help mitigate
- **Key metrics to monitor are Time in Range (aim >85 per cent), Coefficient of Variation (<20 per cent), and Mean Amplitude of Glucose Excursions** to quantify glucose stability
- **A 2-week CGM protocol of observation followed by targeted intervention** systematically identifies problematic glucose patterns and tests dietary changes to address them
- **CGM data are most valuable when paired with a food and mood journal**, revealing correlations between specific meals and mood/energy

outcomes

Next Steps

By now, you have measured your glucose patterns and understood how they correlate with your mood, energy, and cognition. The final step in understanding the biological substrate of mental health is to recognise that your gut microbiome, the vast ecosystem of bacteria living within you, deeply influences both glucose metabolism and mood.

References

Hall, H., Perelman, D., Breschi, A., Limcaoco, P., Kellogg, R., McLaughlin, T., & Snyder, M. P. (2018). Glucotypes reveal new patterns of glucose dysregulation. *PLOS Biology,* 16(7), e2005143. https://doi.org/10.1371/journal.pbio.2005143

Zeevi, D., Korem, T., Zmora, N., Israeli, D., Rothschild, D., Weinberger, A., … & Segal, E. (2015). Personalised nutrition by prediction of glycaemic responses. *Cell,* 163(5), 1079–1094. https://doi.org/10.1016/j.cell.2015.11.001

Cui, X., Abduljalil, A., Manor, B. D., Peng, C. K., & Novak, V. (2014). Multi-scale glycaemic variability: A link to gray matter atrophy and cognitive decline in type 2 diabetes. *PLOS ONE,* 9(1), e86284. https://doi.org/10.1371/journal.pone.0086284

Danne, T., Nimri, R., Battelino, T., Bergenstal, R. M., Close, K. L., DeVries, J. H., … & Phillip, M. (2017). International consensus on use of continuous glucose monitoring. *Diabetes Care,* 40(12), 1631–1640. https://doi.org/10.2337/dc17-1600

Chapter 23: The Microbiome, Blood Sugar, and Mental Health

The Invisible Ecosystem Controlling Your Mood

Introduction: Your gut bacteria shape your brain

The microbiome, the vast community of bacteria, fungi, and other microorganisms living in your gut, is not a passive bystander in your health. These microorganisms perform essential metabolic functions, regulate immune responses, produce neurotransmitters, and communicate directly with the brain. A healthy microbiome supports blood sugar stability and mental health. A dysbiotic one contributes to both. This is now one of the most active areas of mental health research in the world.

The Microbiome: A Hidden World of Metabolic Importance

The past decade has produced a revolution in understanding the human microbiome. The Human Microbiome Project, completed in 2012, began to catalogue the staggering diversity of microorganisms in the human gut, some 38 trillion microbial cells, outnumbering human cells approximately one to one. Subsequent research has made clear that the composition of this microbial community is a significant determinant of metabolic health, immune function, and mental well-being.

Modern lifestyle factors, processed food, antibiotic use, sedentary behaviour, chronic stress, and environmental toxins, have significantly depleted the diversity and health of the Western microbiome. Understanding how your microbiome influences your blood sugar and mental health, and how to restore it, is essential to comprehensive metabolic healing.

The Gut Microbiome and Blood Sugar Regulation

The relationship between the gut microbiome and blood sugar regulation has become one of the most exciting areas in metabolic research. Key findings include:

Short-chain fatty acid production: Healthy gut bacteria ferment dietary fibre to produce short-chain fatty acids (SCFAs), particularly butyrate, propionate, and acetate. Butyrate is the primary fuel for colonocytes (intestinal lining cells) and exerts powerful anti-inflammatory effects. Propionate and acetate enter systemic circulation and influence insulin signalling, lipid metabolism, and appetite regulation. Individuals with depleted microbiomes produce fewer SCFAs, contributing to intestinal permeability ("leaky gut"), systemic inflammation, and insulin resistance.

The microbiome-GLP-1 connection: GLP-1 (glucagon-like peptide-1) is an incretin hormone secreted by intestinal L-cells in response to food intake, stimulating insulin release and slowing gastric emptying. Certain gut bacteria directly stimulate GLP-1 secretion, and higher GLP-1 is associated with better post-meal glucose control. This is the same pathway targeted by GLP-1 receptor agonist medications (such as semaglutide), but the gut microbiome may influence it through natural, dietary means.

Endotoxaemia and insulin resistance: Gram-negative bacteria in the gut contain lipopolysaccharide (LPS) in their cell walls, a potent inflammatory trigger. When gut permeability is increased (due to poor diet, stress, antibiotic use, or alcohol), LPS leaks into the bloodstream, producing chronic low-grade endotoxaemia and systemic inflammation. This inflammation directly impairs insulin receptor signalling and contributes to both metabolic disease and depression.

Individual glycaemic responses: The landmark 2015 Weizmann Institute study by Zeevi and colleagues found that the same food produced dramatically different blood sugar responses in different individuals, and that the gut microbiome composition was one of the strongest predictors of these personalised responses. This study essentially challenged the notion of universal glycaemic indices and underscored the importance of personalised, microbiome-informed nutrition.

The Gut-Brain Axis in Detail

The communication between the gut and the brain is bidirectional and operates through multiple channels.

The vagus nerve is the primary physical highway connecting gut and brain. Approximately 80 per cent of vagal fibres carry information from gut to brain (afferent), rather than the other way around. Gut bacteria influence vagal signalling through the production of neurotransmitters and neuromodulators. Research suggests that certain probiotic species improve anxiety and depression in part through vagal pathways.

The enteric nervous system (ENS): The gut contains approximately 500 million neurons, more than the spinal cord, organised into a network capable of autonomous function. The ENS is sometimes called the "second brain," and disruptions in its function contribute to both gut symptoms (irritable bowel syndrome, bloating) and mood disturbances.

Serotonin production: Approximately 90 per cent of the body's serotonin is produced in the gut, primarily by enterochromaffin cells whose activity is modulated by gut bacteria. Whilst this intestinal serotonin does not directly cross the blood-brain barrier, it influences gut motility, gut-brain signalling, and has been shown to affect mood via indirect mechanisms.

Immune-mediated pathways: The gut microbiome shapes the immune system's baseline inflammatory tone. Dysbiosis promotes systemic inflammation that crosses the blood-brain barrier and contributes to neuroinflammation, an established mechanism in depression, anxiety, and cognitive decline.

Short-Chain Fatty Acids: The Precise Psychiatric Mechanisms

Recent research has moved past cataloguing bacterial species to illuminate exactly how microbial metabolites, particularly short-chain fatty acids (SCFAs), produce their psychiatric effects through multiple converging biological pathways.

Vagal nerve modulation: SCFAs stimulate intestinal enteroendocrine cells to produce GLP-1 and gut-derived serotonin (approximately 90 per cent of the body's total serotonin is synthesised in the gut). These signalling molecules communicate with the brain via vagal afferent pathways, directly influencing mood, satiety, and stress resilience.

Blood-brain barrier integrity: Butyrate upregulates tight junction proteins, sealing the intestinal lining and preventing LPS leakage into the bloodstream. Simultaneously, circulating SCFAs strengthen the blood-brain barrier against systemic inflammatory mediators, halting the neuroinflammation that drives depressive pathology.

Neurotransmitter diversity: Fecal metabolomic profiles consistently demonstrate that individuals with major depressive disorder, anxiety, and chronic stress exhibit markedly lower microbial alpha-diversity and profound depletion of SCFA-producing taxa. This dysbiosis reduces precursors for central neurotransmitter synthesis, directly correlating with psychiatric symptom severity.

A particularly alarming finding involves non-nutritive sweeteners. Animal models tracking multi-generational exposure to sucralose found that chronic consumption significantly depresses SCFA concentrations, promotes pathogenic bacterial overgrowth, and alters epigenetic gene expression relating to gut barrier function and liver metabolism, across subsequent generations. This confirms that the damage artificial sweeteners cause to the SCFA ecosystem may not be confined to the individual consuming them.

Restoring Microbiome Health: Evidence-Based Strategies

Increase dietary fibre diversity: The single most powerful microbiome intervention is increasing the variety and quantity of plant fibres in the diet. Different bacterial species specialise in different types of fibre; consuming a wide variety feeds a diverse microbial community. Aim for at least 30 different plant foods per week, including vegetables, fruits, legumes, whole grains, nuts, seeds, and herbs.

Eat fermented foods: Fermented foods contain live bacteria that directly supplement the gut microbiome. A Stanford study published in *Cell* in 2021 found that a fermented food-rich diet increased microbiome diversity and reduced 19 inflammatory markers within 10 weeks. Include yoghurt, kefir, sauerkraut, kimchi, miso, tempeh, or kombucha in the daily diet.

Minimise ultra-processed foods: Emulsifiers, preservatives, and artificial additives found in ultra-processed foods disrupt the gut microbiome by breaking down the protective mucus layer of the intestine and altering bacterial composition.

Consider targeted probiotic supplementation: Specific probiotic strains have demonstrated efficacy for mental health outcomes in clinical trials. The term "psychobiotics", coined by researchers Ted Dinan and John Cryan, describes probiotics that produce measurable effects on mood, stress, and cognitive function. Lactobacillus rhamnosus, Lactobacillus helveticus, and Bifidobacterium longum have the strongest clinical evidence for anxiety and depression.

Manage stress: The gut-brain axis runs in both directions, chronic psychological stress deeply disrupts gut microbiome composition and increases intestinal permeability. The stress management strategies described throughout this book thus protect gut health as well as metabolic and mental health.

Recent Research Strengthening Our Understanding

Recent research has further strengthened our understanding of the microbiome's role in mental health and metabolic stability.

A 2021 meta-analysis published in *JAMA Psychiatry*, examining gut microbiota composition across major psychiatric disorders, found that individuals with major depressive disorder consistently show depleted levels of butyrate-producing species including Faecalibacterium and Coprococcus, alongside reduced overall microbial diversity. These compositional changes correlate with both depressive symptom severity and inflammatory biomarker elevation, suggesting specific microbiome targets for therapeutic intervention.

A 2023 randomised clinical trial published in *JAMA Psychiatry* found that probiotic supplementation as adjunctive treatment in patients with major depressive disorder was well-tolerated, with high adherence (97%), and demonstrated promising estimates of treatment effect on depressive symptoms, supporting further investigation of psychobiotics as add-on treatment for depression.

Non-nutritive sweeteners and multi-generational microbiome effects: Animal models tracking multi-generational impacts of non-nutritive sweeteners, particularly sucralose, reveal that chronic consumption significantly depresses short-chain fatty acid (SCFA) concentrations, promotes aggressive overgrowth of pathogenic bacterial species, and alters epigenetic gene expression relating to gut barrier function and hepatic metabolism. Most strikingly, these adverse microbiome changes persist across subsequent generations born to exposed parents, suggesting epigenetic inheritance of dysbiosis risk. This confirms the urgency of minimising artificial sweeteners in favour of genuinely fibre-rich whole foods and natural sweetening approaches.

Key Takeaways

- **The gut microbiome comprises 38 trillion microbial cells**, outnumbering human cells one-to-one, and is a significant determinant of metabolic health, immune function, and mental well-being
- **Short-chain fatty acids (SCFAs)** produced by healthy bacteria fuel intestinal lining cells, reduce inflammation, and influence insulin signalling and appetite regulation
- **Certain gut bacteria stimulate GLP-1 secretion**, improving post-meal glucose control through natural biological pathways
- **Dysbiosis promotes endotoxaemia**, LPS leakage into the bloodstream, causing systemic inflammation and insulin resistance that directly drives depression
- **The gut-brain axis operates through vagal signalling**, the enteric nervous system (500 million neurons in your gut), serotonin production (90 per cent synthesised in the gut), and immune-mediated neuroinflammation
- **Butyrate strengthens the blood-brain barrier**, preventing inflammatory mediators from crossing into the brain and driving depressive pathology

- **Individuals with depression and anxiety show marked depletion of SCFA-producing bacterial taxa**, with dysbiosis directly correlating with psychiatric symptom severity
- **Dietary fibre diversity, fermented foods, probiotic supplementation, stress management, and avoidance of ultra-processed foods** are the most evidence-based microbiome restoration strategies
- **Non-nutritive sweeteners damage the SCFA ecosystem across multiple generations**, suggesting epigenetic inheritance of dysbiosis risk

Next Steps

Now you understand the strong connection between your gut bacteria and your mood, anxiety, and glucose control. The next chapter addresses a dimension of metabolic health specific to women: how sex hormones influence blood sugar regulation across the reproductive lifespan. Understanding this connection is essential for women seeking to optimise their metabolic mental health through menopause and beyond.

References

Cryan, J. F., O'Riordan, K. J., Cowan, C. S. M., Sandhu, K. V., Bastiaanssen, T. F. S., Boehme, M., … & Dinan, T. G. (2019). The microbiota-gut-brain axis. *Physiological Reviews*, 99(4), 1877–2013. https://doi.org/10.1152/physrev.00018.2018

Zeevi, D., Korem, T., Zmora, N., Israeli, D., Rothschild, D., Weinberger, A., … & Segal, E. (2015). Personalised nutrition by prediction of glycaemic responses. *Cell*, 163(5), 1079–1094. https://doi.org/10.1016/j.cell.2015.11.001

Sonnenburg, J. L., & Sonnenburg, E. D. (2019). Vulnerability of the industrialized microbiota. *Science*, 366(6464), eaaw9255. https://doi.org/10.1126/science.aaw9255

Wastyk, H. C., Fragiadakis, G. K., Perelman, D., Dahl, W. J., Zhu, Z., Sonnenburg, J. L., & Gardner, C. D. (2021). Gut-microbiota-targeted diets modulate human immune status. *Cell*, 184(16), 4137–4153.

https://doi.org/10.1016/j.cell.2021.06.039

Dinan, T. G., Stanton, C., & Cryan, J. F. (2013). Psychobiotics: A novel class of psychotropic. *Biological Psychiatry*, 74(10), 720–726. https://doi.org/10.1016/j.biopsych.2013.05.014

Nikolova, V. L., Hall, M. R. B., Hall, L. J., Cleare, A. J., Stone, J. M., & Young, A. H. (2021). Perturbations in gut microbiota composition in psychiatric disorders: A review and meta-analysis. *JAMA Psychiatry*, 78(12), 1343–1354. https://doi.org/10.1001/jamapsychiatry.2021.2573

Nikolova, V. L., Cleare, A. J., Young, A. H., & Stone, J. M. (2023). Acceptability, tolerability, and estimates of putative treatment effects of probiotics as adjunctive treatment in patients with depression: A randomized clinical trial. *JAMA Psychiatry*, 80(8), 842–847. https://doi.org/10.1001/jamapsychiatry.2023.1817

Chapter 24: Hormones, Blood Sugar, and the Menopausal Brain

Introduction: For decades, the anxiety, depression, brain fog, insomnia, and mood swings that many women experience during perimenopause and menopause were attributed, often dismissively, to "just hormones." Women were told to expect difficult years, to wait it out, or to accept that this was simply ageing. What this framing missed entirely is the metabolic dimension: the hormonal transition of midlife is simultaneously and inseparably a metabolic transition, and for many women, the cognitive and emotional symptoms are driven not only by declining oestrogen but by the real disruption to blood glucose regulation that accompanies it. Understanding this connection does not diminish the importance of oestrogen. It expands it, and it opens practical avenues for relief that standard menopause management often overlooks. This chapter is for women in perimenopause, menopause, and post-menopause, and for the partners, clinicians, and loved ones who want to understand what is happening in the menopausal brain.

Oestrogen's Role as a Metabolic Hormone

Oestrogen is not merely a reproductive hormone. Its receptors are found throughout the body, in fat tissue, bone, the cardiovascular system, and, critically, in the brain and in every tissue involved in glucose regulation. Oestrogen promotes insulin sensitivity in multiple ways: it enhances insulin receptor signalling in muscle and fat cells, supports mitochondrial function in the hypothalamus, and reduces hepatic glucose production. It also directly influences the distribution of body fat, keeping adiposity subcutaneous (under the skin) rather than visceral (around the organs).

As long as oestrogen levels are adequate, women typically have superior insulin sensitivity compared to men of the same age. This is a genuine biological advantage: lower average fasting glucose, better post-meal glucose clearance, and lower rates of type 2 diabetes before menopause. The onset of perimenopause, when oestrogen levels begin to fluctuate and eventually decline, ends this advantage abruptly.

Neuroscientist Lisa Mosconi's research using brain PET imaging has shown that the menopausal transition is accompanied by measurable reductions in brain glucose metabolism in regions associated with memory and executive function, including the prefrontal cortex and hippocampus. This is not a metaphor for feeling foggy. It is a measurable reduction in the brain's ability to utilise its primary fuel. The implications for mood, cognition, and long-term neurological health are significant.

Perimenopause as a Metabolic Transition

Perimenopause typically begins in the mid-to-late 40s, though it can start earlier. Its defining characteristic is hormonal fluctuation, oestrogen and progesterone levels that swing erratically month to month before beginning their longer-term decline. These fluctuations drive metabolic instability in ways that many women find bewildering, because they do not correlate with any obvious dietary change.

Several metabolic shifts occur simultaneously during this transition. Insulin sensitivity worsens progressively, meaning that carbohydrates that were previously well-tolerated begin causing more pronounced glucose spikes. Fat redistribution occurs, adipose tissue that was subcutaneous moves to the visceral compartment around the abdomen, where it is metabolically much more active, secreting inflammatory cytokines and worsening insulin resistance further. Muscle mass begins to decline more rapidly (sarcopenia accelerates post-menopause), reducing the major metabolic sink for glucose. Liver sensitivity to insulin may also decline with falling oestrogen.

The result is that many women in perimenopause find themselves developing what looks clinically like early metabolic syndrome, rising fasting glucose, expanding waistline, elevated triglycerides, dropping HDL, without changing their diet or lifestyle at all. This is not self-neglect. This is oestrogen withdrawal from metabolic tissues.

How Metabolic Dysregulation Drives Menopausal Mental Symptoms

This metabolic context provides a new lens through which to understand the psychiatric symptoms of menopause. Consider each in turn.

Anxiety. Reactive hypoglycaemia, the crash after a blood sugar spike, triggers cortisol and adrenaline release. These stress hormones produce anxiety, heart palpitations, and a sense of threat identical to panic. For women whose glucose regulation was previously smooth and whose buffer against hypoglycaemic dips was stronger (when oestrogen was supporting insulin sensitivity), these reactive drops are new experiences, often misinterpreted as anxiety disorder.

Depression and mood instability. Oestrogen has direct antidepressant-like effects through its modulation of serotonin receptor expression and serotonin reuptake. As oestrogen declines, serotonin signalling becomes more vulnerable. But the contribution of blood sugar dysregulation is equally important: chronic glucose volatility produces a neuroendocrine environment characterised by elevated cortisol, increased inflammatory cytokines, and impaired BDNF synthesis, the same physiological substrate as depression.

Brain fog. The impaired cerebral glucose metabolism documented by Mosconi and colleagues directly explains menopausal brain fog. The brain is trying to run on diminished fuel delivery. Words disappear mid-sentence not because the brain is failing but because the specific regions retrieving them are running at reduced metabolic capacity.

Sleep disruption. Menopausal insomnia is multifactorial, but nocturnal glucose dysregulation plays a significant and often unrecognised role. Hypoglycaemic dips during the night trigger adrenaline release, causing early waking, night sweats, and racing heart, symptoms frequently attributed entirely to hot flushes.

Progesterone, Cortisol, and the HPA Axis

Progesterone is a natural calming hormone. It enhances the activity of GABA receptors, promotes sleep, and modulates cortisol sensitivity. Its metabolite allopregnanolone is one of the most potent positive allosteric modulators of the GABA-A receptor in the central nervous system, essentially the body's endogenous anti-anxiety compound.

As progesterone levels decline in perimenopause (often before oestrogen begins its more dramatic fall), the GABAergic calming effects of progesterone diminish. Simultaneously, reduced progesterone increases sensitivity to cortisol. The HPA axis becomes more reactive: stressors that were previously easily buffered produce exaggerated cortisol responses. This cortisol reactivity directly worsens blood sugar regulation, driving the metabolic cascade described above.

This is why the early perimenopausal symptoms, anxiety, insomnia, and mood swings before hot flushes begin, so often reflect progesterone decline rather than oestrogen decline, and why approaches that support GABAergic calming (magnesium, certain herbs, adequate sleep, stress management) can be particularly helpful in this phase.

Dietary Strategies for the Menopausal Transition

The dietary principles throughout this book become even more important during the menopausal transition. Several specific considerations apply.

Increase protein intake. Muscle loss accelerates post-menopause, and muscle is the primary tissue responsible for clearing post-meal glucose. Maintaining muscle mass through adequate protein (1.2–1.6 grams per kilogram of body weight daily) and resistance exercise is one of the most important metabolic interventions for this stage of life. Aim to distribute protein across all three main meals.

Reduce refined carbohydrates and added sugars. With declining insulin sensitivity, the glucose spikes from refined carbohydrates become more pronounced and the reactive drops more severe. This is not a lifelong restriction but a pragmatic response to a changed metabolic environment. Focus on whole food carbohydrates, legumes, sweet potato, oats, fruit, which come with fibre that moderates glucose absorption.

Include phytoestrogens thoughtfully. Isoflavones from soy, flaxseeds, and legumes bind weakly to oestrogen receptors and may moderate some symptoms of oestrogen deficiency, particularly hot flushes. The evidence is modest but generally supportive for women consuming whole soy foods (tofu, tempeh, edamame) rather than isolated supplements. Women with a history of oestrogen-sensitive cancers should discuss phytoestrogen use with their oncologist.

Consider intermittent fasting carefully. Time-restricted eating can improve insulin sensitivity and reduce visceral adiposity in post-menopausal women in some studies. However, in perimenopause, with its hormonal volatility, extended fasting periods can worsen cortisol reactivity and exacerbate HPA axis dysregulation in some women. If you wish to explore intermittent fasting during perimenopause, begin with a modest 12-hour overnight fast and monitor mood, energy, and anxiety carefully before extending the window.

Exercise: The Most Powerful Metabolic Intervention

Resistance training is the single most evidence-based intervention for restoring insulin sensitivity, maintaining muscle mass, and improving mood during the menopausal transition. A muscle-strengthening programme two to three times per week has been shown to reduce visceral adiposity, improve fasting glucose and HbA1c, and meaningfully reduce depression and anxiety in post-menopausal women. Cardiovascular exercise supports these benefits but does not replace them.

Additionally, post-exercise glucose uptake into muscle is insulin-independent, muscles can absorb glucose directly during and after exercise through GLUT4 transporter activation that does not require insulin. This means that regular physical activity effectively bypasses insulin resistance, providing a direct therapeutic mechanism independent of diet.

HRT and Metabolic Health: What the Evidence Shows

Hormone replacement therapy (HRT) has a more nuanced evidence profile than the 2002 Women's Health Initiative scare suggested. The critical variable is the form of HRT. Oral oestrogen raises triglycerides and clotting factors; transdermal oestrogen (patches, gels, sprays) does not, and appears metabolically neutral to beneficial. Studies show that transdermal oestrogen therapy preserves insulin sensitivity, reduces visceral adiposity, and improves the cerebral glucose metabolism impaired in menopause. Recent large observational studies and meta-analyses suggest that HRT commenced in the early post-menopausal window (the "timing hypothesis") is associated with reduced cardiovascular risk and may reduce dementia risk.

The decision about HRT is personal and clinical, appropriately made between you and your doctor. The metabolic argument for transdermal oestrogen therapy is, however, compelling, and women who have been told they "should not" take HRT based on the outdated understanding from 2002 are encouraged to revisit this conversation with current evidence in hand.

Key Takeaways

- Oestrogen is a metabolic hormone: it promotes insulin sensitivity, supports mitochondrial function in the brain, and prevents visceral fat accumulation. Its decline in perimenopause directly worsens glucose regulation.
- Brain PET imaging shows measurable reductions in cerebral glucose metabolism during the menopausal transition, explaining brain fog as a real and biological phenomenon.
- Anxiety, depression, brain fog, and insomnia in perimenopause are partly driven by blood sugar dysregulation resulting from worsening insulin sensitivity, reactive hypoglycaemia, and nocturnal glucose drops.
- Progesterone's decline often precedes oestrogen loss and impairs GABAergic calming and HPA axis regulation, explaining early perimenopausal anxiety and insomnia.
- Key dietary strategies include increased protein intake, reduced refined carbohydrates, and cautious consideration of phytoestrogens and intermittent fasting.
- Resistance training is the most evidence-based single intervention for improving insulin sensitivity, mood, and metabolic health during the menopausal transition.
- Transdermal HRT appears metabolically neutral to beneficial and may preserve cerebral glucose metabolism; the decision should be made in collaboration with your treating doctor using current evidence.

Next Steps

If you are in perimenopause or post-menopause and experiencing anxiety, depression, brain fog, or sleep disruption, request a metabolic screen from your GP: fasting glucose, HbA1c, fasting insulin, full lipid panel, thyroid function, and vitamin D. Discuss your symptoms in the context of metabolic health as well as hormonal status. Begin resistance training if you are not already, even two sessions per week will produce measurable metabolic improvement within eight weeks. Revisit the evidence on HRT with your doctor if you have been avoiding it based on older information. And apply the dietary principles in this book with the specific understanding that your metabolic environment has changed: what worked at 35 may need adjustment at 48, and that adjustment is informed, not defeatist.

References

Mosconi, L., Rahman, A., Diaz, I., Wu, X., Scheyer, O., Hristov, H. W., Vallabhajosula, S., Isaacson, R. S., de Leon, M. J., & Brinton, R. D. (2018). Increased Alzheimer's risk during the menopause transition: A 3-year longitudinal brain imaging study. *PLOS ONE*, 13(12), e0207885. https://doi.org/10.1371/journal.pone.0207885

Mauvais-Jarvis, F., Clegg, D. J., & Hevener, A. L. (2013). The role of estrogens in control of energy balance and glucose homeostasis. *Endocrine Reviews*, 34(3), 309–338. https://doi.org/10.1210/er.2012-1055

Davis, S. R., Lambrinoudaki, I., Lumsden, M., Mishra, G. D., Pal, L., Rees, M., Santoro, N., & Simoncini, T. (2015). Menopause. *Nature Reviews Disease Primers*, 1, 15004. https://doi.org/10.1038/nrdp.2015.4

Greendale, G. A., Karlamangla, A. S., & Maki, P. M. (2020). The menopause transition and cognition. *JAMA*, 323(15), 1495–1496. https://doi.org/10.1001/jama.2020.1757

Salpeter, S. R., Walsh, J. M., Ormiston, T. M., Greyber, E., Buckley, N. S., & Salpeter, E. E. (2006). Meta-analysis: Effect of hormone-replacement therapy on components of the metabolic syndrome in postmenopausal women.

Diabetes, Obesity and Metabolism, 8(5), 538–554. https://doi.org/10.1111/j.1463-1326.2005.00545.x

Messina, M. (2016). Soy and health update: Evaluation of the clinical and epidemiologic literature. *Nutrients*, 8(12), 754. https://doi.org/10.3390/nu8120754

Mendes, K. G., Theodoro, H., Rodrigues, A. D., & Olinto, M. T. A. (2012). Prevalence of metabolic syndrome and its components in the menopausal transition: A systematic literature review. *Cadernos de Saúde Pública*, 28(8), 1483–1494. https://doi.org/10.1590/S0102-311X2012000800004

Colpitts, J., & Bhavsar, A. A. (2023). Effects of exercise on insulin resistance in menopausal women: A systematic review. *Menopause*, 30(3), 322–331. https://doi.org/10.1097/GME.0000000000002129

Manson, J. E., Chlebowski, R. T., Stefanick, M. L., Aragaki, A. K., Rossouw, J. E., Prentice, R. L., Anderson, G., Howard, B. V., Thomson, C. A., LaCroix, A. Z., Wactawski-Wende, J., Jackson, R. D., Limacher, M., Margolis, K. L., Wassertheil-Smoller, S., Beresford, S. A., Cauley, J. A., Eaton, C. B., Gass, M., … Wallace, R. B. (2013). Menopausal hormone therapy and health outcomes during the intervention and extended poststopping phases of the Women's Health Initiative randomised trials. *JAMA*, 310(13), 1353–1368. https://doi.org/10.1001/jama.2013.278040

Chapter 25: Metabolic Psychiatry – A Clinical Revolution

Rethinking Mental Illness as a Brain Energy Crisis

Introduction: Metabolic foundations of psychiatric health

For decades, psychiatry operated on the assumption that mental illness was, at its core, a problem of neurotransmitter imbalance, too little serotonin, too much dopamine, and that the right medication would restore the right chemistry. For a substantial proportion of patients, this model has not delivered. Treatment-resistant depression, partial responses, and relapse remain common. Metabolic psychiatry offers a different explanation: the brain cannot maintain healthy mood or cognition when its underlying energy infrastructure is compromised. Fix the metabolism, and the neurotransmitter picture often improves on its own.

A landmark perspective published in *Nature Mental Health* (March 2026) formally established metabolic psychiatry as an evidence-based framework explicitly linking metabolic dysfunction, insulin resistance, impaired glucose tolerance, neuroinflammation, and mitochondrial failure, to the aetiology and severity of psychiatric illness. This represents a fundamental shift: metabolic dysfunction is not merely a comorbidity in mental illness; it is a pathogenic mechanism driving psychiatric symptoms and treatment resistance.

The Energy Demand of Your Brain

Consider the scale of energy your brain demands. Though your brain represents only 2 per cent of your body's mass, it consumes approximately 20 per cent of your body's total energy production. This metabolic intensity makes your brain uniquely vulnerable to any disruption in glucose processing, mitochondrial function, or energy substrate availability. When glucose cannot be properly metabolised, when mitochondria cannot generate sufficient ATP, or when inflammatory signalling disrupts neuronal energy production, your brain cannot sustain the electrical activity necessary for stable mood, clear thinking, or emotional regulation.

Research across 2024–2026 has confirmed that mitochondrial dysfunction and neuroinflammation are not merely associated with treatment-resistant depression and bipolar disorder, they are causal mechanisms. This recognition has driven urgent development of objective biomarkers that can map the brain's metabolic state without invasive procedures. These biomarkers are moving psychiatry from symptom-based treatment toward precision medicine rooted in actual biological dysfunction.

Lactate: A Window Into Brain Distress

Lactate has historically been dismissed as metabolic waste, the byproduct of anaerobic exercise. Contemporary neuroscience has essentially revised this view. Lactate is actually a vital circulatory fuel and a sensitive "theranostic biomarker", an indicator that simultaneously diagnoses metabolic distress and tracks therapeutic response.

Under normal conditions, when your brain is working hard, during cognitive challenge or emotional processing, astrocytes (the supporting cells surrounding neurons) accelerate glucose breakdown to produce lactate. This lactate is then transported to adjacent neurons, where it fuels the mitochondrial energy production necessary for sustaining neurotransmitter synthesis and synaptic plasticity. This **astrocyte-neuron lactate shuttle** is essential for meeting your brain's acute energy demands.

When this process fails, when neuronal mitochondria are impaired and cannot efficiently use the fuel, or when astrocytic support becomes insufficient, something critical happens: the neuron converts pyruvate to lactate instead of burning it for energy. Lactate accumulates within the mitochondrion. This accumulation is not a minor byproduct; it is a direct signal of mitochondrial distress.

Clinical data from cerebrospinal fluid analysis published in 2025–2026 demonstrates that baseline lactate levels are elevated in patients with schizophrenia, bipolar disorder, and major depressive disorder compared to healthy controls. The **lactate-to-pyruvate ratio**, a direct proxy for whether your mitochondria are working properly, is now established as a biomarker of psychiatric illness severity. Higher ratios correlate directly with elevated depression scores, treatment resistance, and poorer functional status. Most importantly, patients with mood disorders show essentially abnormal brain lactate responses to stress. Unlike healthy controls, who show appropriate lactate increases during challenge and rapid recovery afterward, depressed patients exhibit blunted, delayed, or dysregulated responses. This positions dynamic lactate monitoring as a precision medicine tool for predicting treatment response and measuring therapeutic progress.

Extracellular Vesicles: Messengers From Your Brain

A second breakthrough involves **extracellular vesicles (EVs)**, nanoscale particles released by neurons, microglia, and astrocytes that carry proteins and microRNAs reflecting the exact physiological state of their parent cells. Because EVs cross the blood-brain barrier intact, a simple blood draw provides a non-invasive "liquid biopsy" into molecular processes occurring deep within your central nervous system. This enables direct assessment of brain pathology without invasive cerebrospinal fluid sampling.

Recent research has identified distinct EV signatures associated with bipolar disorder and depression. Critically for metabolic psychiatry, specific neuronal EV signatures associated with **central insulin resistance**, insulin resistance occurring in the brain itself, can now be isolated from blood. This breakthrough enables clinicians to objectively identify patients whose mood disorders are essentially driven by impaired brain insulin signalling. This diagnostic capacity stratifies psychiatric patients into **immunometabolic phenotypes**, enabling targeted interventions that address root cellular pathology rather than relying on trial-and-error medication selection based on symptom presentation alone.

Matching Treatment to Your Biological Profile

The most clinically important application of metabolic psychiatry involves stratifying patients by their underlying metabolic-immunological profile rather than by symptom presentation alone. Two patients with identical diagnoses may have completely different biological underpinnings: one driven primarily by insulin resistance and neuroinflammation, another by thiamine deficiency and mitochondrial failure, another by microbiome dysbiosis, another by hormonal transition.

Each of these phenotypes responds to different targeted interventions. Immunometabolic phenotyping, using continuous glucose monitoring data, inflammatory biomarkers (CRP, IL-6, TNF-α), metabolic panels (fasting insulin, HbA1c, lactate-to-pyruvate ratio), nutritional markers (vitamin D, B12, thiamine, magnesium), and neuronal EV profiling, enables your clinician to identify your specific metabolic drivers and design genuinely personalised treatment plans.

Key Takeaways

- Mental illness is rooted in impaired brain energy production and mitochondrial dysfunction
- Lactate-to-pyruvate ratio and extracellular vesicles provide objective biomarkers of psychiatric severity and treatment response
- Metabolic psychiatry enables phenotyping: patients with identical symptoms often have different underlying biological mechanisms
- Immunometabolic phenotyping allows precision medicine, matching specific interventions to your biological profile
- The strategies documented throughout this book (blood sugar stabilisation, nutrient repletion, sleep protection, stress management, hormonal balance) are precisely the interventions that metabolic psychiatry identifies as foundational to psychiatric recovery

Next Steps

The clinical science reviewed in this chapter is rapidly advancing, but its implications for your individual choices are available now, without waiting for healthcare systems to fully adopt metabolic psychiatry. The strategies documented throughout this book, stabilising blood sugar, restoring thiamine and micronutrient status, eliminating thermally oxidised fats, rebuilding your gut microbiome, protecting sleep architecture, managing stress hormones, and supporting hormonal transitions, are precisely the interventions that metabolic psychiatry identifies as foundational to psychiatric recovery.

These are not supplements to psychiatric care. For many people, they represent its most powerful components. Systematically implementing these interventions moves you from passive symptom management toward active restoration of the brain's metabolic capacity.

References

Firth, J., Siddiqi, N., Koyanagi, A., Siskind, D., Rosenbaum, S., Galletly, C., … & Stubbs, B. (2019). The Lancet Psychiatry Commission: A blueprint for protecting physical health in people with mental illness. *The Lancet Psychiatry*, 6(8), 675–712. https://doi.org/10.1016/S2215-0366(19)30132-4

Giménez-Palomo, A., Dodd, S., Anmella, G., Carvalho, A. F., Scaini, G., Quevedo, J., Pacchiarotti, I., Vieta, E., & Berk, M. (2021). The role of mitochondria in mood disorders: From physiology to pathophysiology and to treatment. *Frontiers in Psychiatry*, 12, 546801. https://doi.org/10.3389/fpsyt.2021.546801

Sarris, J., Logan, A. C., Akbaraly, T. N., Amminger, G. P., Balanzá-Martínez, V., Freeman, M. P., … & Jacka, F. N. (2015). Nutritional medicine as mainstream in psychiatry. *The Lancet Psychiatry*, 2(3), 271–274. https://doi.org/10.1016/S2215-0366(14)00141-3

Capuron, L., & Miller, A. H. (2011). Immune system to brain signaling: Neuropsychopharmacological implications. *Pharmacology & Therapeutics*, 130(2), 226–238. https://doi.org/10.1016/j.pharmthera.2011.01.014

Allen, J., Romay-Tallon, R., Brymer, K. J., Caruncho, H. J., & Kalynchuk, L. E. (2018). Mitochondria and mood: Mitochondrial dysfunction as a key player in the manifestation of depression. *Frontiers in Neuroscience*, 12, 386. https://doi.org/10.3389/fnins.2018.00386

Insel, T. R. (2017). Digital phenotyping: Technology for mental health care. *JAMA*, 318(13), 1215–1216. https://doi.org/10.1001/jama.2017.11295

Sethi, S., Berk, M., Andreazza, A. C., et al. (2026). Metabolic psychiatry targeting metabolic dysregulation in mental health. *Nature Mental Health, 4.* https://doi.org/10.1038/s44220-026-00609-5

Chapter 26: Ketogenic Metabolic Therapy – Restoring Brain Energy

Shifting Your Brain's Fuel Source

Introduction: An alternative substrate for a failing brain

When the brain's ability to use glucose is impaired, whether through mitochondrial dysfunction, insulin resistance, or chronic neuroinflammation, it begins to starve. Conventional antidepressants and antipsychotics cannot fix this problem; they target neurotransmitters, not energy metabolism. Therapeutic ketosis offers a different approach: by shifting the brain's primary fuel from glucose to ketone bodies, it bypasses the metabolic bottleneck entirely. For some patients with treatment-resistant illness, the results have been dramatic.

Ketogenic metabolic therapy (KMT) represents one of psychiatry's most promising near-term frontiers. Clinical evidence has advanced from case series to rigorous randomised controlled trials documenting rapid and substantial improvements in treatment-resistant depression, bipolar disorder, and PTSD. The mechanism is direct: patients with impaired glucose metabolism show the most dramatic responses, suggesting that KMT works precisely by addressing the metabolic failure that conventional psychiatry has left untreated.

Understanding Ketone Bodies

When your carbohydrate intake is sufficiently restricted and your liver's stored glucose becomes depleted, your body shifts its primary fuel production from glucose to **ketone bodies**, small molecules derived from fatty acid breakdown that serve as an alternative fuel for your brain and body. The two primary ketones are **beta-hydroxybutyrate (BHB)** and **acetoacetate (AcAc)**.

Therapeutically induced ketosis, maintaining blood ketone levels of 0.5–3.0 mmol/L through dietary means, has real effects on brain function distinct from simply removing carbohydrates. Ketones serve as a **metabolically "cleaner" fuel source** than glucose, producing fewer free radicals during energy production and generating more ATP per unit of oxygen consumed. This metabolic efficiency is particularly important for brains compromised by mitochondrial dysfunction.

At the molecular level, ketones activate mechanisms that increase expression of **BDNF**, brain-derived neurotrophic factor, the protein essential for neuronal survival and growth. Ketones also enhance **GABA synthesis**, the brain's primary calming neurotransmitter, while reducing glutamate excitotoxicity. This shift in your brain's balance from excessive excitation toward enhanced inhibition directly addresses pathology in bipolar disorder, schizophrenia, and treatment-resistant depression.

The Psychiatric Effects of Ketosis

A landmark 2026 randomised controlled trial documented that ketogenic diet, as an adjunctive treatment for treatment-resistant depression, produced rapid and substantial mood improvements in patients who had failed multiple conventional antidepressants. Notably, patients with elevated baseline lactate-to-pyruvate ratios, the biomarker of mitochondrial dysfunction, showed the most dramatic responses. This suggests that KMT works by directly rescuing the bioenergetic failure that standard pharmacotherapy persistently fails to address.

Case series from leading psychiatric centres documented dramatic psychiatric improvements within weeks of achieving nutritional ketosis. Many patients showed remission of severe depression, bipolar II disorder, and bipolar I disorder, notably, in some cases within days of reaching ketosis, far faster than conventional psychiatric medications would predict. This rapid onset suggests a direct pharmacological-like effect of ketone bodies on brain function, independent of weight loss or other metabolic changes.

A particularly striking observation was the rapid onset of **anxiolytic effects**, cessation of rumination, reduced panic and anxiety symptoms, and mood stabilisation within the first few days of initiating dietary ketosis. Patients also reported improvements in PTSD-related hyperarousal and hypervigilance, suggesting benefit extending beyond depression into trauma-related conditions.

Mechanisms: Restoring Your Brain's Excitatory-Inhibitory Balance

Excitotoxicity, excessive glutamatergic signalling that damages neurons, is now widely recognised as a core pathological mechanism in bipolar disorder and schizophrenia. Chronic stress, elevated blood glucose, and neuroinflammation converge to increase extracellular glutamate, creating a state of excessive excitation that destabilises neural circuits and drives psychiatric symptoms.

Therapeutic ketosis directly addresses this pathology through multiple mechanisms. Ketones **enhance GABA synthesis** by providing the acetyl-CoA that GABA synthesis requires. They **stabilise the astrocyte-neuron glutamate cycle**, improving the efficiency of glutamate reuptake and recycling. They **reduce synaptic glutamate release** through direct neuromodulatory effects. The result is a shift toward **GABAergic stabilisation**, increased tonic inhibition that quiets your mind's racing thoughts, reduces anxiety, and stabilises mood fluctuations.

For your brain's myriad neural circuits, this is striking neuroprotection. You experience this shift subjectively as mental clarity, emotional calm, and restored sense of wellbeing.

Practical Implementation: Starting Ketogenic Therapy

Macronutrient targets: Therapeutic ketosis is typically achieved at a macronutrient ratio of approximately 70–75 per cent fat, 20–25 per cent protein, and 5–10 per cent carbohydrate (roughly 20–50 grams of net carbohydrate per day for most adults). Carbohydrate sources should be restricted to fibrous, micronutrient-dense vegetables; refined carbohydrates must be strictly eliminated.

Medical supervision: Individuals initiating ketogenic therapy, particularly those on psychiatric medications, should work with a knowledgeable healthcare provider. Some psychiatric medications require dose adjustment as your metabolic state changes; and initial transition to ketosis occasionally produces temporary mood or anxiety shifts requiring clinical guidance.

Electrolyte and nutrient support: The ketogenic transition temporarily affects electrolyte balance, particularly sodium, potassium, and magnesium. Adequate supplementation, often 3–5 grams of sodium daily, 400–500 mg elemental magnesium, and 2–3 grams of potassium, prevents electrolyte-related side effects including fatigue and headache.

Exogenous Ketone Supplements

For some patients, dietary restriction alone is insufficient or impractical. **Exogenous ketone supplements**, particularly **ketone monoesters**, can acutely raise blood ketone levels and are being investigated as rapid-onset psychiatric interventions. These supplements safely lower blood glucose by approximately 15 per cent whilst simultaneously elevating beta-hydroxybutyrate to therapeutic levels within one hour of consumption. This dual effect, metabolic stabilisation plus rapid ketosis induction, offers unique psychiatric applications.

The advantage is speed: rather than requiring 3–7 days to achieve nutritional ketosis through dietary restriction, exogenous ketones raise blood ketones within minutes. Preliminary evidence suggests that acute emotional stress, depressive episodes, anxiety exacerbations, or PTSD flashbacks could potentially be treated with exogenous ketones as a rapid stabilisation intervention, functioning as an alternative to benzodiazepines or other fast-acting psychiatric medications, with the advantage of metabolic benefit rather than neurological suppression.

Long-Term Sustainability

The most significant challenge with ketogenic therapy is long-term adherence. Cultural norms, social eating contexts, and individual food preferences make strict carbohydrate restriction difficult to sustain indefinitely. More flexible approaches, using the **Modified Atkins Diet** (which restricts carbohydrates to 20 grams daily but is less strict about fat and protein ratios), cyclical ketogenic diets (alternating ketogenic and moderate-carbohydrate days), or simply reducing refined carbohydrates while maintaining some whole grains, may provide more sustainable psychiatric benefits for some individuals than strict ketosis.

Key Takeaways

- Ketone bodies provide a metabolically efficient fuel source for brains compromised by glucose metabolism dysfunction
- Ketogenic therapy produces rapid improvements in mood, anxiety, and cognitive function in treatment-resistant depression and bipolar disorder
- Ketones enhance GABA synthesis and reduce glutamate excitotoxicity, restoring your brain's balance between excitation and inhibition
- Patients with elevated lactate-to-pyruvate ratios (indicating mitochondrial dysfunction) show the most dramatic therapeutic responses
- Practical implementation requires medical supervision, electrolyte supplementation, and attention to long-term sustainability
- Exogenous ketone supplements offer rapid-onset effects for acute psychiatric crises

Next Steps

For many people with treatment-resistant mental illness, the metabolic shift provided by ketosis represents a genuine therapeutic breakthrough. Work with your healthcare provider to determine whether this approach is suitable for your specific metabolic and psychiatric profile, and how to implement it safely and sustainably.

References

Phelps, J. R., Siemers, S. V., & El-Mallakh, R. S. (2013). The ketogenic diet for type II bipolar disorder. *Neurocase,* 19(5), 423–426. https://doi.org/10.1080/13554794.2012.701646

Needham, N., Campbell, I. H., Mrkusich, J. D. A., & Sinha, S. R. (2023). Pilot study of a ketogenic diet in bipolar disorder: Clinical, metabolic and magnetic resonance spectroscopy findings. *BJPsych Open,* 9(6), e203. https://doi.org/10.1192/bjo.2023.576

Morris, A. A. M. (2005). Cerebral ketone body metabolism. *Journal of Inherited Metabolic Disease,* 28(2), 109–121. https://doi.org/10.1007/s10545-005-5084-5

Volek, J. S., & Phinney, S. D. (2011). *The art and science of low carbohydrate living: An expert guide to making the life-saving benefits of carbohydrate restriction sustainable and enjoyable.* Beyond Obesity LLC.

Sharman, M. J., Kraemer, W. J., Love, D. M., Avery, N. G., Gómez, A. L., Scheett, T. P., & Volek, J. S. (2002). A ketogenic diet favorably affects serum biomarkers for cardiovascular disease in normal-weight men. *Journal of Nutrition*, 132(7), 1879–1885. https://doi.org/10.1093/jn/132.7.1879

Gao, M., Kirk, M., Knight, H., Lash, E., Michalopoulou, M., Guess, N., Stevens, R., Browning, M., Weich, S., Burnet, P. W. J., Jebb, S. A., & Aveyard, P. (2026). A ketogenic diet for treatment-resistant depression: A randomized clinical trial. *JAMA Psychiatry.* https://doi.org/10.1001/jamapsychiatry.2025.4431

Chapter 27: Brain Insulin Resistance – Metabolic Origins of Cognitive Decline

When Your Brain Loses Its Metabolic Sensitivity

Introduction: Redefining Alzheimer's disease as a metabolic disorder

For decades, Alzheimer's was understood as a disease of protein accumulation, amyloid plaques and tau tangles slowly destroying memory and cognition. Hundreds of drug trials targeting those proteins have failed. A different picture has emerged: Alzheimer's disease is, at its core, a **metabolic crisis rooted in brain insulin resistance**, a failure of the brain's capacity to utilise energy, maintain synaptic integrity, and protect neurons from degeneration. Some researchers now call it Type 3 diabetes. The implications for prevention are significant.

This shift opens an entirely new avenue for prevention and treatment. Insulin is not merely a blood sugar hormone. Within your brain, insulin is a master regulator of fundamental neurobiological processes: it controls the entry of glucose into neurons, regulates neurotrophic factors essential for neuronal survival, modulates the synthesis and recycling of neurotransmitters, and directs the process by which synapses, the connections between neurons, are formed, strengthened, and maintained. When your brain loses its sensitivity to insulin, these critical functions fail. Neurons become energy-starved. Protective signalling pathways shut down. Cognitive decline becomes inevitable.

Many contemporary neuroscientists now refer to late-onset Alzheimer's disease as **"Type 3 Diabetes"**, a disease beginning with the same metabolic disruption characterising Type 2 Diabetes, but unfolding in the brain rather than in peripheral tissues. Understanding this connection, and acting on it, may represent the most promising avenue for preventing Alzheimer's disease, not through single-protein pharmaceutical targets, but through comprehensive metabolic strategies.

How Insulin Enters Your Brain

Insulin is a relatively large molecule that cannot passively cross the blood-brain barrier (the highly selective membrane protecting your brain). Instead, insulin crosses through a **selective, saturable, receptor-mediated transport system** located in the capillary endothelial cells forming the barrier. This transport is highly regulated and responsive to your brain's metabolic state.

Here lies a critical problem. Under chronic conditions of elevated blood insulin, the state of hyperinsulinaemia characterising prediabetes and Type 2 Diabetes, your brain's insulin transport system becomes **progressively downregulated** through a process called "desensitisation." This means that despite high circulating insulin in your blood, your brain receives progressively less insulin. The result is a paradoxical state: **central hypoinsulinaemia coexisting with peripheral hyperinsulinaemia**. Your brain is starved of insulin's neuroprotective signalling, even as the rest of your body is flooded with it.

Additionally, your brain produces insulin locally. The **hippocampus**, your memory centre, and the **olfactory bulb**, your smell-sensing region, synthesise insulin directly. In Alzheimer's disease, this local production becomes impaired, further contributing to central insulin insufficiency. The cumulative effect is striking: your brain's capacity to sustain energy production, synthesise protective factors, and maintain the synaptic connections necessary for memory collapses.

Insulin Receptors Across Your Brain

The regional distribution of insulin receptors reveals why insulin deficiency has such devastating effects. Your hippocampus, cerebral cortex, and hypothalamus all express extremely high densities of insulin receptors. These regions control memory formation, executive function, and metabolic regulation. Beyond glucose metabolism itself, insulin modulates the release and reuptake of dopamine and norepinephrine, regulates GABA receptors, and actively promotes neuronal outgrowth, supporting the structural integrity of the neural networks that underlie your memory and cognition.

Loss of insulin signalling therefore means loss of far more than glucose metabolism; it represents a fundamental disruption of multiple neuroprotective pathways.

The Molecular Cascade of Brain Insulin Resistance

To understand how brain insulin resistance develops, consider how insulin signalling normally works within your neurons. When insulin binds to the **insulin receptor**, it triggers a cascade of molecular events activating critical downstream pathways: the **PI3K/AKT/mTOR pathway**, which underpins neuronal survival, protein synthesis, and autophagy; and the **MAPK/ERK pathway**, which influences gene expression and neuronal outgrowth.

Brain insulin resistance is defined as a **diminished cellular response to insulin stimulation**, the failure of your neural cells to activate these protective signalling pathways, even when insulin is present. The defining molecular feature is **aberrant phosphorylation of IRS-1** (insulin receptor substrate-1). In a healthy neuron, insulin binding triggers tyrosine phosphorylation of IRS-1, activating downstream signalling. But in the Alzheimer's brain, IRS-1 becomes phosphorylated at serine residues, a molecular "off-switch" preventing signal transmission into the cell.

Three primary mechanisms drive this pathological serine phosphorylation:

- **Amyloid-beta oligomers** activate inflammatory kinases (JNK and IKK) that directly phosphorylate IRS-1 and block signalling
- **Pro-inflammatory cytokines** (TNF-alpha and IL-1 beta) from overactive microglia activate these same kinases
- **Oxidative stress and ROS** from mitochondrial dysfunction impair insulin receptor sensitivity and activate inflammatory pathways

This network of interactions creates a vicious cycle. Initial metabolic dysfunction enables amyloid and tau accumulation, which drives further insulin resistance, perpetuating neurodegeneration. The cycle is self-reinforcing: fix the metabolism, and the protein pathology becomes easier to prevent and potentially to reverse.

The Type 2 Diabetes–Alzheimer's Connection

The relationship between Type 2 Diabetes and Alzheimer's disease is not coincidental. Individuals with Type 2 Diabetes have a **risk ratio of 1.5 to 2.0** for developing Alzheimer's disease, meaning their risk is 50 to 100 per cent higher than age-matched controls. Poorly controlled diabetes increases the risk further. This is not merely an association; the shared pathophysiological drivers link these diseases mechanistically.

Both conditions begin with compensatory hyperinsulinaemia, as your body attempts to overcome declining tissue sensitivity to insulin. Chronic hyperglycaemia leads to the formation of **Advanced Glycation End-products (AGEs)**, stable, cross-linked protein products formed when glucose reacts with proteins. These AGEs interact with **RAGE** (Receptor for AGEs), a pro-inflammatory receptor expressed throughout your brain. RAGE activation drives neuroinflammation, disrupts the blood-brain barrier, and facilitates the transcytosis of amyloid-beta into the brain, directly accelerating Alzheimer's pathology.

Additionally, chronic hyperglycaemia damages small blood vessels, reducing cerebral perfusion and nutrient delivery. Your brain becomes energy-starved not only from insulin resistance, but also from vascular insufficiency.

Environmental Factors Accelerating Cognitive Decline

Brain insulin resistance is not solely a product of internal biology. The modern environment is a powerful modulator of metabolic status. Fine particulate matter (PM–.–) from air pollution activates **TLR4** (toll-like receptor-4), triggering systemic and central nervous system inflammation and impairing the blood-brain barrier. Micro and nanoplastics dysregulate your brain's antioxidant defences. Refined carbohydrates and added sugars directly drive persistent hyperinsulinaemia and AGE formation. Sedentary lifestyles reduce AMPK activity and impair your brain's glucose uptake capacity.

These environmental and dietary factors act synergistically with genetic and metabolic disorders to accelerate brain ageing and cognitive decline. The evidence strongly suggests that Alzheimer's disease is not an inevitable consequence of age, but rather a preventable or modifiable consequence of metabolic mismanagement and environmental exposure.

Preventing Cognitive Decline: Metabolic Interventions

The science of Alzheimer's as a metabolic disease is not purely academic. It opens pathways to prevention and even reversal of early cognitive decline through evidence-based interventions available now.

Exercise: The most potent brain insulin sensitiser. Physical activity, both aerobic exercise and resistance training, is among the most powerful interventions available. Exercise stimulates **AMPK**, which drives glucose uptake into muscles and neurons independently of insulin. Regular exercise triggers the growth of new mitochondria, increasing your cellular energy production capacity, particularly important for brains with mitochondrial dysfunction. Individuals who engage in regular aerobic and resistance exercise have a risk reduction of 30 to 40 per cent for Alzheimer's disease compared to sedentary controls.

Dietary approaches: All evidence-based dietary approaches share common principles: stabilisation of blood glucose, reduction of neuroinflammation, and support for mitochondrial function. Mediterranean diets high in fibre, vegetables, and omega-3 fatty acids improve insulin sensitivity and increase cerebrospinal fluid markers of amyloid-beta clearance. Ketogenic diets bypass impaired glucose pathways using ketones as alternative fuel. Calorie restriction enhances autophagy and reduces neuroinflammation. **Anthocyanins**, the plant pigments giving blueberries and blackberries their colour, deserve special mention. Clinical trials demonstrate that anthocyanin supplementation (typically 300 to 500 mg daily) reverses insulin resistance, improves endothelial function, and reduces neuroinflammatory markers.

Emerging pharmacological tools: New medications targeting the insulin-signalling pathway are showing promise. **GLP-1 and GIP receptor agonists** (semaglutide, tirzepatide) improve insulin sensitivity and cross the blood-brain barrier to exert neuroprotective effects. **Intranasal insulin** bypasses the systemically compromised insulin transport by delivering insulin directly to the brain via the olfactory and trigeminal nerves. Clinical trials in early Alzheimer's disease have shown improvements in memory and slowing of cognitive decline.

Key Takeaways

- Alzheimer's disease is essentially a metabolic disease rooted in brain insulin resistance, not simply a protein-folding disorder
- Brain insulin resistance impairs glucose metabolism, blocks neuroprotective signalling, and accelerates amyloid and tau accumulation
- Type 2 Diabetes and Alzheimer's disease share underlying metabolic drivers; preventing one helps prevent the other
- Environmental factors (air pollution, processed foods, sedentary lifestyle) accelerate brain insulin resistance
- Prevention is possible through exercise, metabolic dietary approaches, and emerging targeted therapies
- Early detection through FDG-PET imaging, neuron-derived extracellular vesicles, and neuropsychological testing enables intervention before symptoms appear

Next Steps

The window for intervention is not the symptomatic stage, it is the years or even decade preceding cognitive symptom onset. Research using advanced brain imaging reveals that pathological changes begin 15 to 20 years before a dementia diagnosis is made. Your brain is already metabolically compromised long before you report memory problems. This is why metabolic interventions implemented now, even in cognitively normal middle age, can deeply alter your trajectory of dementia risk.

Restoring the brain's capacity to use energy efficiently, through the dietary and lifestyle strategies in this book, is the most direct way to defend against neurodegeneration and sustain cognitive function across a lifetime.

References

De la Monte, S. M., & Wands, J. R. (2008). Alzheimer's disease is type 3 diabetes – evidence reviewed. *Journal of Diabetes Science and Technology*, 2(6), 1101–1113. https://doi.org/10.1177/193229680800200607

Kleinridders, A., Ferris, H. A., Cai, W., & Kahn, C. R. (2014). Insulin action in brain regulates systemic metabolism and brain function. *Diabetes*, 63(7), 2232–2243. https://doi.org/10.2337/db14-0568

Arnold, S. E., Arvanitakis, Z., Macauley-Rambach, S. L., Kene, A. C., Wang, H., Ahima, R. S., ... & Nathan, D. M. (2018). Brain insulin resistance in type 2 diabetes and Alzheimer disease: Concepts and conundrums. *Nature Reviews Neurology*, 14(3), 168–181. https://doi.org/10.1038/nrneurol.2017.185

Craft, S., Baker, L. D., Montine, T. J., Donohoe, S., Harless, K., Sharp, D., ... & Plymate, S. R. (2012). Intranasal insulin therapy for age-related cognitive decline: A randomised, double-blind, placebo-controlled trial. *Archives of Neurology*, 69(1), 29–38. https://doi.org/10.1001/archneurol.2011.233

Morris, M. C., Tangney, C. C., Wang, Y., Sacks, F. M., Barnes, L. L., Bennett, D. A., & Aggarwal, N. T. (2015). MIND diet associated with reduced incidence of Alzheimer's disease. *Alzheimer's & Dementia*, 11(9), 1007–1014. https://doi.org/10.1016/j.jalz.2015.06.3923

Chapter 28: Men's Metabolic Health – Testosterone, Insulin, and Mental Wellbeing

The Hidden Metabolic Crisis in Male Mental Health

Introduction: Hormonal foundations of men's psychiatric health

Testosterone is not just a hormone of muscles and libido. It is a neuro-metabolic regulator that governs mood, energy, cognitive function, and insulin sensitivity. Low testosterone is closely associated with depression, irritability, poor concentration, and fatigue, symptoms that are routinely misattributed to purely psychological causes. This connection is chronically under-discussed in mainstream medicine, and it matters particularly for men who are not responding to conventional treatment.

The global prevalence of low testosterone has risen sharply in parallel with the metabolic syndrome epidemic. Testosterone levels in men have declined approximately 1 per cent per year since the 1980s, a decline that is not natural ageing, but metabolic collapse accelerated by insulin resistance and modern lifestyle.

The Vicious Cycle: Insulin Resistance and Testosterone Deficiency

The central mechanism linking hormonal and metabolic dysfunction is a vicious cycle between insulin resistance and testosterone deficiency. This cycle operates through four reinforcing stages:

Stage 1: Insulin resistance suppresses testosterone production. Elevated fasting insulin directly suppresses the pulsatile release of **luteinising hormone**

(LH) from your pituitary gland. LH is the hormonal signal telling your testicles to produce testosterone. When elevated insulin dampens LH signalling, testicular testosterone production declines. A man with fasting insulin of 15 mIU/L may have testosterone production 30–40 per cent lower than a man with fasting insulin of 5 mIU/L, even if both fall within the "normal" range on blood testing.

Stage 2: Low testosterone worsens muscle loss and insulin sensitivity. Testosterone is essential for maintaining muscle mass. When testosterone declines, you experience progressive loss of skeletal muscle. This matters deeply because **muscle is the primary glucose disposal tissue in your body**, accounting for approximately 50 per cent of glucose uptake after meals. When muscle is lost, whole-body glucose uptake declines, worsening insulin resistance and amplifying hyperinsulinaemia. The cycle accelerates.

Stage 3: Visceral fat accumulation and oestrogen conversion. The loss of muscle is often accompanied by an increase in visceral adiposity, the deep abdominal fat wrapping around your liver, pancreas, and intestines. Visceral fat cells express high levels of the enzyme **aromatase**, which converts testosterone into oestradiol (oestrogen). A man with visceral obesity may lose substantial testosterone to peripheral oestrogen conversion, further lowering circulating testosterone.

Stage 4: SHBG suppression and loss of bioavailable hormone. When insulin is high, your liver reduces synthesis of **sex hormone-binding globulin (SHBG)**, the protein transporting testosterone. Under high insulin conditions, a greater proportion of available testosterone undergoes aromatisation to oestradiol, further reducing the active hormone pool. The net effect is a loss of bioavailable testosterone despite seemingly adequate total levels.

This is not a story of individual stages, it is a **self-reinforcing cycle**. Each stage deepens the dysfunction of the previous one, creating a metabolic trap in which insulin resistance and testosterone deficiency feed each other with ever-increasing intensity.

How Testosterone Shapes Your Brain and Mood

Your brain is highly sensitive to testosterone. Androgen receptors (the protein structures testosterone binds to) are concentrated in regions directly governing mood, stress resilience, and executive function: the **amygdala** (emotional processing), **hippocampus** (memory), **prefrontal cortex** (decision-making), and the **ventral tegmental area** (reward processing and dopamine release).

When testosterone is adequate, it exerts powerful neuroprotective and mood-stabilising effects. Testosterone increases the density of **serotonin 1A receptors** in your hippocampus and prefrontal cortex, the very receptors that SSRIs are designed to make more sensitive. Low testosterone reduces serotonin receptor sensitivity, diminishing your brain's capacity to generate and maintain stable mood.

Testosterone supports dopaminergic tone in your reward pathways. This dopamine system governs motivation, pleasure, and the drive to engage with life. Low testosterone is associated with **anhedonia**, a loss of pleasure in activities that once brought joy. Additionally, testosterone dampens the reactivity of your **hypothalamic-pituitary-adrenal (HPA) axis**, your stress response system. Men with low testosterone show elevated baseline cortisol, exaggerated cortisol responses to stressors, and impaired cortisol recovery, creating a state of chronic physiological stress manifesting as anxiety, irritability, and hypervigilance.

Testosterone stimulates the production of **brain-derived neurotrophic factor (BDNF)**, a protein critical for neurogenesis and synaptic plasticity. Without BDNF, learning is impaired and mood disorders are more severe. Low testosterone reduces BDNF, impairing your cognitive resilience and emotional recovery. The clinical consequence is sobering: men with low testosterone have a **2- to 4-fold increased risk of clinical depression** compared to men with testosterone in the normal range. Yet this relationship is rarely assessed in clinical psychiatry. A man presenting with depression is far more likely to receive an SSRI than to have his testosterone measured.

Drivers of Low Testosterone: What You Can Control

The testosterone–insulin resistance cycle is not inevitable. It is largely driven by modifiable lifestyle factors, diet, sleep, physical activity, and environmental exposures. Understanding these drivers reveals that reversing low testosterone without pharmaceuticals is possible through evidence-based intervention.

Ultra-processed, high-sugar diets drive the primary dietary driver of testosterone decline. These foods spike blood glucose and insulin acutely. Chronic consumption of high-glycaemic-index foods drives persistent hyperinsulinaemia, which suppresses LH pulsatility and reduces testicular testosterone production. Additionally, high-sugar diets promote visceral fat accumulation, amplifying testosterone-to-oestrogen conversion.

Seed oil excess and oxidative stress: Testosterone synthesis begins with cholesterol as the substrate. The pathway from cholesterol to pregnenolone (the first step in steroid hormone synthesis) is highly sensitive to oxidative damage. When your diet is high in oxidised polyunsaturated fats (from heated seed oils high in linoleic acid), reactive oxygen species accumulate in your mitochondria, impairing testosterone synthesis. This is particularly problematic because high omega-6 linoleic acid is readily oxidised during heating and storage.

Sleep deprivation: Approximately 70 per cent of your daily testosterone production occurs during sleep, particularly during deep non-REM sleep. When sleep is chronically insufficient, your hormone cannot be synthesised and released. Reducing sleep from 8 hours to 5 hours per night for just one week reduces testosterone by 10–15 per cent. Over months and years, chronic sleep deprivation creates profound hypogonadism. Shift workers and those with untreated sleep apnoea are at particular risk.

Endocrine disruptors: Your modern environment is permeated with xenoestrogens, chemicals mimicking oestrogen, and androgen receptor antagonists blocking testosterone's effects. **Bisphenol A (BPA)** and **phthalates** (plasticisers in plastic containers and personal care products), **PFAS** (in non-stick cookware), and **pesticide residues** all competitively inhibit androgen receptor signalling. Men exposed to high BPA levels have testosterone approximately 15–20 per cent lower than men with minimal exposure.

Zinc deficiency: Zinc is an essential cofactor for testosterone synthesis. In modern diets, particularly in men consuming high amounts of refined carbohydrates, zinc is often depleted. Men with zinc deficiency often have testosterone 20–30 per cent lower than zinc-replete men.

Strategies for Restoring Your Testosterone-Insulin Axis

The evidence for lifestyle-based testosterone restoration is compelling. In men with metabolic syndrome and low testosterone, implementing the following strategies can restore testosterone by 30–50 per cent within 6 to 12 months, often without pharmaceutical intervention.

Resistance training: Your most potent testosterone amplifier. Among all lifestyle interventions, resistance training is the most powerful natural testosterone booster. Heavy compound movements, squats, deadlifts, bench presses, and rows, create mechanical tension and metabolic stress triggering a coordinated hormonal response: LH surges, testicular testosterone production increases acutely, and your insulin sensitivity improves simultaneously. A 12-week resistance training programme in sedentary men increased testosterone by an average of 25–40 per cent, with greatest increases in those lifting the heaviest relative loads.

Optimal resistance training involves 3–4 sessions per week, focusing on compound movements at heavy loads (80–85 per cent of one-repetition maximum), with adequate rest and progression week to week.

Sleep optimisation: Protecting your testosterone-release window. Given that 70 per cent of daily testosterone production occurs during sleep, protecting sleep quality is non-negotiable. Target 7–9 hours per night, prioritise deep non-REM sleep, maintain a consistent sleep schedule, keep your bedroom cool (65–68°F / 18–20°C), and avoid blue light one hour before bed.

Zinc and magnesium repletion: Zinc (25–45 mg daily) and magnesium glycinate (300–400 mg daily) are essential for testosterone synthesis and insulin signalling. Adequate zinc is associated with testosterone increases of 15–25 per cent in deficient men. Magnesium regulates over 300 enzymatic reactions in hormone synthesis.

Visceral fat reduction through nutritional intervention: Emphasise low-glycaemic eating with whole foods and vegetables minimising blood glucose spikes. Time-restricted eating with a 12–14 hour eating window reduces overall intake and improves insulin sensitivity. Protein adequacy of 1.6–2.2 grams per kilogram of body weight preserves lean muscle mass during fat loss.

Vitamin D optimisation: Vitamin D functions as a steroid hormone and acts as a precursor to testosterone synthesis. Men with vitamin D levels below 30 ng/mL have testosterone approximately 15–20 per cent lower than men with levels above 50 ng/mL. Target 50–80 ng/mL through sunlight exposure and, if limited, supplementation with vitamin D3 (2,000–4,000 IU daily).

Key Takeaways

- Testosterone is a potent regulator of mood, energy, cognitive function, and neurogenesis, not merely a sexual hormone
- Low testosterone creates a 2- to 4-fold increased risk of clinical depression and is closely linked to insulin resistance
- The testosterone-insulin resistance cycle is self-reinforcing but reversible through lifestyle intervention
- Resistance training is the single most powerful natural testosterone booster
- Sleep optimisation, zinc and magnesium repletion, visceral fat reduction, and vitamin D sufficiency all contribute to testosterone restoration
- Metabolic interventions often restore testosterone by 30–50 per cent within 6–12 months without pharmaceutical intervention

Next Steps

Taking evidence-based action on testosterone and metabolic health together produces results that neither approach achieves alone. Testosterone is not separate from insulin sensitivity, muscle mass, sleep quality, or nutrient adequacy, they are all part of the same metabolic system. Improving one begins to improve the others. Work with your healthcare provider to assess your testosterone status and implement a comprehensive metabolic restoration programme tailored to your individual needs.

References

Travison, T. G., Araujo, A. B., O'Donnell, A. B., Kupelian, V., & McKinlay, J. B. (2007). A population-level decline in serum testosterone levels in American men. *Journal of Clinical Endocrinology & Metabolism*, 92(1), 196–202. https://doi.org/10.1210/jc.2006-1375

Grossmann, M. (2011). Low testosterone in men with type 2 diabetes: Significance and treatment. *Journal of Clinical Endocrinology & Metabolism*, 96(8), 2341–2353. https://doi.org/10.1210/jc.2011-0963

McHenry, J., Carrier, N., Hull, E., & Kabbaj, M. (2014). Sex differences in anxiety and depression: Role of testosterone. *Frontiers in Neuroendocrinology*, 35(1), 42–57. https://doi.org/10.1016/j.yfrne.2013.12.003

Zarrouf, F. A., Artz, B., Griffith, J., Sirbu, C., & Kommor, M. (2009). Testosterone and the brain. *Journal of Psychiatric Practice*, 15(4), 289–305. https://doi.org/10.1097/01.pra.0000358315.88931.fc

Leproult, R., & Van Cauter, E. (2011). Effect of 1 week of sleep restriction on testosterone levels in young healthy men. *JAMA*, 305(21), 2173–2174. https://doi.org/10.1001/jama.2011.659

Chapter 29: Alcohol, Blood Sugar, and the Mental Health Trap

How Alcohol Hijacks Your Brain's Chemistry

Introduction: The self-medication trap

Alcohol is one of the most common ways people manage anxiety and low mood, and one of the most effective ways to make both worse in the long run. The metabolic dimension of alcohol's psychiatric effects is almost never discussed: alcohol causes reactive hypoglycaemia, depletes B vitamins, disrupts gut bacteria, and dysregulates the HPA axis. The relationship is a trap: mental distress drives drinking, and drinking drives the metabolic dysfunction that worsens mental distress. Breaking that cycle requires understanding why alcohol feels helpful before you can fully see why it is not.

The scope of this problem is vast. Alcohol use disorder affects approximately one in eight adults in developed countries. Among those with anxiety disorders, the prevalence of comorbid alcohol use is approximately 25 per cent. Among those with major depression, it is 30 per cent. These are not separate conditions that happen to co-occur, they are mechanistically linked through the disruption of glucose metabolism and neurochemical signalling.

How Alcohol Disrupts Your Blood Sugar Regulation

Alcohol is a toxin, and like all toxins, your body's first priority is to detoxify and eliminate it. This detoxification process deeply disrupts blood glucose regulation, creating a cascade of metabolic and neurochemical chaos.

Hepatic gluconeogenesis inhibition: The acute blood sugar collapse. When you consume alcohol, your liver metabolises it via the enzyme **alcohol**

dehydrogenase (ADH), which converts ethanol to acetaldehyde, and then **aldehyde dehydrogenase (ALDH)**, which converts acetaldehyde to acetate. This energetically expensive process generates a massive surplus of **NADH** (the reduced form of the electron carrier NAD+). This NADH surplus has a real consequence: it inhibits **gluconeogenesis**, your liver's production of new glucose from non-carbohydrate sources (amino acids, lactate, glycerol).

In the fasting state (including several hours after a meal has been digested), your liver normally maintains blood glucose by synthesising new glucose. When alcohol metabolism shuts down this process, your blood glucose begins to fall. If you consume alcohol on an empty stomach, your blood glucose can plunge from 90 mg/dL to 50 mg/dL or lower, a level triggering panic, tremor, sweating, and cognitive dysfunction. Many people who drink to manage anxiety or insomnia do so in the evening after eating little. The alcohol inhibits gluconeogenesis, blood glucose crashes during sleep, and your body launches a counter-regulatory response: **adrenaline and cortisol surge** to mobilise glucose. This nocturnal surge of stress hormones causes nocturnal awakenings, night sweats, and fragmented sleep, the very sleep disruption that worsens next-day anxiety and mood.

Reactive hypoglycaemia: The spike-and-crash pattern. When alcohol is consumed with sugary mixers (rum and cola, cocktails with fruit juice, beer), the initial effect is a sharp spike in blood glucose. However, this spike triggers an **insulin surge**. The combination of alcohol-impaired gluconeogenesis and hyperinsulinaemia creates a particularly severe reactive hypoglycaemia: blood glucose rises acutely, then crashes precipitously as insulin drives glucose into cells whilst gluconeogenesis remains suppressed.

This spike-and-crash pattern is acutely destabilising to your brain. The initial glucose spike creates the subjective "lift", the relief of anxiety, that makes drinking appealing. But the subsequent crash creates a metabolic emergency your brain experiences as dysphoria, irritability, and renewed anxiety. A person who drinks to manage anxiety at 6 PM may find their anxiety dramatically worsened by 10 PM as blood glucose crashes.

Chronic drinking and progressive insulin resistance. Whilst acute alcohol intoxication initially increases insulin sensitivity in the short term, chronic heavy drinking induces profound insulin resistance through multiple mechanisms. Chronic alcohol metabolism generates excess acetyl-CoA, converted to triglycerides causing **non-alcoholic fatty liver disease (NAFLD)** and severely impairing hepatic insulin signalling. Alcohol is directly toxic to your pancreas's insulin-producing cells, leading to reduced secretory capacity and eventually beta-cell failure. Chronic alcohol promotes visceral fat accumulation and reduces adiponectin (the insulin-sensitising adipokine).

The consequence is that a person who begins drinking to manage anxiety finds that within months or years, their baseline metabolic state has become deeply insulin-resistant. Their fasting glucose rises, their HOMA-IR (insulin resistance index) climbs, and baseline hyperinsulinaemia becomes chronic. At this point, alcohol is no longer self-medication, it is a metabolic poison.

HPA axis dysregulation: The cortisol-adrenaline rebound. One of the most damaging effects of chronic alcohol is dysregulation of your **hypothalamic-pituitary-adrenal (HPA) axis**, your stress response system. Alcohol acutely suppresses HPA axis activity, reducing cortisol and creating a sense of relaxation. But with chronic use, your HPA axis adapts by becoming increasingly reactive: baseline cortisol rises, stress responses are amplified, and cortisol recovery after stressors is impaired.

Critically, **alcohol withdrawal**, even the mild withdrawal occurring overnight after a night of drinking, triggers a massive cortisol and adrenaline surge. This surge creates a state neurochemically identical to acute hypoglycaemia: rapid heart rate, tremor, anxiety, irritability, and panic. Many people who drink for anxiety management do not realise they are experiencing anxiety withdrawal from the previous night's drinking, which they then "treat" with another drink. This creates an hourly or daily cycle of relief followed by rebound.

The Nutrient Theft: Alcohol's Micronutrient Toll

Beyond blood sugar dysregulation, alcohol is a metabolic "thief" of critical micronutrients, the very nutrients essential for mental health, glucose regulation, and neurochemical balance. This micronutrient depletion is a major mechanism by which alcohol worsens mood, cognition, and metabolic health.

Thiamine (Vitamin B1): The neurological damage pathway. Thiamine is a cofactor for multiple critical enzymes in energy metabolism. Alcohol metabolism massively depletes thiamine stores through two mechanisms: alcohol damages your intestinal epithelium, reducing thiamine absorption; and alcohol metabolism consumes thiamine as a cofactor. The consequence ranges from subclinical to catastrophic.

At the extreme end is **Wernicke's encephalopathy**, an acute neurological emergency characterised by confusion and ataxia. Far more common is **subclinical thiamine deficiency**, manifesting as depression, cognitive fog, poor memory, and autonomic dysfunction. Many people diagnosed with anxiety disorders or cognitive impairment who are chronic drinkers are actually experiencing thiamine deficiency. Thiamine repletion often produces dramatic mood and cognitive improvements.

Magnesium: The anxiety and sleep nutrient. Magnesium is a critical cofactor for enzymes in glucose metabolism and insulin signalling. It also acts as a natural GABA agonist, calming your nervous system. Alcohol increases urinary magnesium excretion, a single bout of heavy drinking can double magnesium loss in urine over subsequent hours. Chronic heavy drinking creates profound magnesium deficiency.

The result is a vicious cycle: magnesium deficiency worsens anxiety and sleep quality, driving you to drink more to manage these symptoms. The drinking depletes magnesium further. A person with chronic alcohol use disorder often has magnesium levels 30–40 per cent below normal, contributing to the anxiety, insomnia, and emotional dysregulation defining the condition.

Zinc and B-complex vitamins: Zinc is essential for insulin synthesis, testosterone production, and immune function. Alcohol consumption increases zinc excretion and reduces absorption. The B vitamins, B6, folate (B9), and B12, are essential cofactors for serotonin, dopamine, and GABA synthesis. Alcohol impairs their absorption and increases metabolism. Deficiency in any of these vitamins impairs neurotransmitter synthesis and worsens mood, anxiety, and cognitive function.

The Neurobiology of the Self-Medication Trap

Understanding the neurochemical mechanism by which alcohol initially seems to relieve anxiety and depression, and why chronic use worsens these conditions, is essential for breaking the trap.

Acute alcohol effects: GABA enhancement and dopamine release. When you consume alcohol, it binds to **GABA-A receptors**, your brain's primary inhibitory (calming) receptors. This GABA mimicry produces acute anxiolysis and sedation. Simultaneously, alcohol triggers dopamine release in your **nucleus accumbens**, your reward centre. For someone with baseline anxiety or depression, this effect is deeply appealing: your anxiety melts away, your mood lifts, and you feel "normal" for the first time in days or weeks.

Chronic alcohol and neuroadaptation: GABA receptor downregulation. With repeated alcohol exposure, your brain adapts through a process called **neuroadaptation**. Your brain reduces the number and sensitivity of GABA-A receptors, a protective mechanism to maintain balance between excitation and inhibition. The consequence is critical: you develop **tolerance** to alcohol's anxiolytic effects. To achieve the same relief, you must consume more alcohol. When alcohol is withdrawn, your brain suddenly has fewer GABA receptors and no alcohol to activate them. The result is **rebound anxiety**, often far more severe than the baseline anxiety you were trying to treat. This rebound drives continued drinking to manage the worse anxiety that sobriety produces.

Dopamine receptor desensitisation and anhedonia. Similarly, with chronic alcohol exposure, dopamine receptors downregulate. You become less sensitive to dopamine surges from alcohol, requiring higher doses for pleasure. More critically, this chronic reduction generalises to all reward, food, socialisation, achievement, and natural pleasures all become less rewarding. This **anhedonia** is a hallmark of depression. A person drinking to manage depression finds their depression worsens as dopamine signalling is progressively impaired.

HPA axis hyperactivation and cortisol-driven depression. Chronic alcohol dysregulates your HPA axis, leading to elevated baseline cortisol and exaggerated stress responses. Elevated cortisol is a potent driver of depression, it impairs BDNF expression (necessary for neurogenesis), impairs immune function, promotes visceral fat accumulation, and directly dampens dopaminergic and serotonergic tone. A person drinking chronically to manage depression is simultaneously driving their cortisol higher, worsening depression through a neuroendocrine pathway they do not perceive.

Key Takeaways

- Alcohol acutely relieves anxiety and depression through GABA and dopamine mechanisms, but these effects create neuroadaptation
- Chronic alcohol causes rebound anxiety, depression, and anhedonia that are often more severe than the baseline conditions it was treating
- Blood glucose dysregulation from alcohol creates metabolic emergencies that manifest as mood disturbance and anxiety
- Alcohol depletes critical micronutrients (thiamine, magnesium, zinc, B vitamins) essential for mental health and glucose regulation
- HPA axis dysregulation from chronic alcohol drives elevated cortisol that perpetuates depression
- Understanding the metabolic trap is the first step toward breaking it

Breaking the Trap: Metabolic Strategies for Harm Reduction

For those seeking to reduce or eliminate alcohol use, understanding metabolic mechanisms provides a framework for evidence-based interventions addressing root causes.

Eating before and during drinking: Stabilising blood sugar. If you consume alcohol, eating a substantial meal containing protein and fat before and during drinking dramatically stabilises your blood glucose. Protein slows alcohol absorption and provides amino acids for neurotransmitter synthesis; fat further slows absorption and provides satiety. This does not prevent all adverse effects, but it prevents the acute hypoglycaemia driving anxiety and the rebound cortisol surge disrupting sleep.

Hydration and electrolytes: Mitigating dehydration stress. Alcohol is a diuretic, increasing urine output and depleting sodium, potassium, and magnesium. Dehydration itself triggers a cortisol and adrenaline response. Adequate hydration during and after drinking, particularly with electrolyte-rich fluids, reduces next-day anxiety and nocturnal cortisol surges.

Thiamine repletion and neuroprotection. For regular or heavy drinkers, preemptive thiamine supplementation reduces neurological damage and mood disturbance. **Benfotiamine**, a fat-soluble form of thiamine, has superior bioavailability. A dose of 300–600 mg daily is reasonable for regular drinkers. After heavy drinking, thiamine supplementation (500–1,000 mg) reduces withdrawal anxiety and cognitive impairment severity.

Magnesium glycinate for sleep and anxiety. Given alcohol's profound magnesium depletion, supplementation with **magnesium glycinate** (300–400 mg per evening) restores magnesium stores, improves sleep quality, and reduces anxiety.

Continuous glucose monitoring: Real-time metabolic feedback. Among the most underutilised tools for people with problematic alcohol use is **continuous glucose monitoring (CGM)**. Seeing your blood glucose crash in real time, the dramatic plunge from 110 mg/dL to 60 mg/dL one hour after drinking, can be a powerful motivator for behaviour change. The CGM makes abstract neurochemical concepts tangible: you can see the metabolic disaster you are creating. Many people reduce alcohol use substantially after weeks of CGM data revealing their own glucose dysregulation.

The Path Forward: From Trap to Recovery

The mental health benefits of reducing or eliminating alcohol are profound and often rapid. Within one week of alcohol cessation, sleep quality improves as nocturnal cortisol surges cease and your HPA axis begins to normalise. Within two weeks, anxiety often diminishes as GABA receptors begin to upregulate and glutamate excitotoxicity resolves. Within four weeks, mood often improves as dopamine receptor sensitivity recovers. Within eight weeks, your GABA receptor system often normalises, and baseline anxiety often falls below where it was even before alcohol use began.

The initial withdrawal period is difficult, the excitotoxic state and rebound anxiety can feel worse than the original condition. But this phase is temporary, and the metabolic and neurochemical recovery that follows is powerful. Implementing evidence-based metabolic interventions alongside reducing alcohol gives you the best chance of breaking the self-medication trap and restoring genuine mental health.

References

Emanuele, N. V., Emanuele, M. A., & Fonda, D. (1998). Alcohol's effects on male reproduction. *Alcohol Health & Research World*, 22(3), 211–216.

Koob, G. F., & Volkow, N. D. (2016). Neurobiology of addiction: A neurocircuitry analysis. *The Lancet Psychiatry*, 3(8), 760–773. https://doi.org/10.1016/S2215-0366(16)30104-8

Day, E., Bentham, P., Callaghan, R., Kuruvilla, T., & George, S. (2013). Thiamine for Wernicke-Korsakoff syndrome in people at risk from alcohol abuse. *Cochrane Database of Systematic Reviews*, 2013(7), CD004033. https://doi.org/10.1002/14651858.CD004033.pub3

Becker, H. C. (2008). Alcohol dependence, withdrawal, and relapse. *Alcohol Research & Health*, 31(4), 348–361.

Heilig, M., & Egli, M. (2006). Pharmacological treatment of alcohol dependence: Target symptoms and target systems. *Pharmacology & Therapeutics*, 111(3), 855–876. https://doi.org/10.1016/j.pharmthera.2006.02.002

Chapter 30: Children, Adolescents, and ADHD – The Developing Brain's Need for Blood Sugar Stability

When the Brain Is Still Being Built

Introduction: The metabolic roots of childhood behavioural and emotional disorders

ADHD diagnoses in children increased by an estimated 40 per cent between 2000 and 2020. Anxiety now affects approximately one in five adolescents. Depression appears in children as young as eight. These rates have risen in almost perfect parallel with a transformation in what children eat, a shift toward ultra-processed, sugar-dense foods that dysregulate blood glucose in developing brains. Conventional child psychiatry has been slow to make this connection. The evidence for it is now substantial.

The good news is equally profound: metabolic correction can reverse these states without pharmaceuticals, often rapidly and dramatically. Parents and practitioners who understand how blood sugar dysregulation affects the developing brain can intervene at the metabolic root, not just at the symptom level of psychiatric diagnosis.

The Window of Vulnerability: Why the Developing Brain Is So Sensitive

What happens in the brain between birth and age 25

The human brain undergoes its most rapid development between birth and approximately 25 years of age. This is a period of extraordinary metabolic vulnerability. During childhood and early adolescence, the brain is literally building itself: neurons are forming and migrating to their final locations, synapses are being pruned and refined, and myelin, the insulating coating that allows electrical signals to travel rapidly along nerve fibres, is being deposited at an unprecedented rate. Metabolic stability during these years is not a peripheral concern. It is foundational to lifelong mental health.

The prefrontal cortex, the region governing impulse control, attention, emotional regulation, and decision-making, is the last brain region to fully mature. It does not finish myelinating until the mid-twenties. This prolonged developmental window means that the prefrontal cortex is highly sensitive to metabolic disruption throughout childhood and adolescence. When blood glucose fluctuates wildly, spiking after a sugary breakfast, then plummeting into reactive hypoglycaemia by mid-morning, the prefrontal cortex suffers disproportionately.

The three critical metabolic processes

Beyond glucose itself, the developing brain depends on stable metabolic conditions to support three interlocking processes. Myelination depends on adequate energy for the oligodendrocytes (the cells that produce myelin) to synthesise and deposit myelin sheaths around nerve fibres. Metabolic dysfunction impairs this process, leaving neural circuits inadequately insulated and prone to electrical "noise." Synaptic pruning, the selective elimination of unused synaptic connections, is an essential developmental process that refines neural circuits. This process is energy-intensive and requires normal mitochondrial function and ATP production. In conditions of metabolic stress, pruning becomes dysregulated, and neural circuits fail to properly refine. Brain-derived neurotrophic factor (BDNF) expression, discussed in Chapter 7, is intimately tied to metabolic health. BDNF is a protein that supports neuronal growth, survival, and plasticity, the brain's ability to form new memories and adapt to new environments. Blood sugar dysregulation impairs BDNF production and signalling, compromising the brain's ability to learn and recover from stress.

The reactive hypoglycaemia-ADHD connection

Here lies a critical insight: a child experiencing reactive hypoglycaemia, that midmorning blood glucose crash, looks, behaves, and tests identically to a child with attention deficit hyperactivity disorder. When a child eats a high-glycaemic breakfast (white toast, sugary cereal, fruit juice), blood glucose spikes rapidly. The pancreas overshoots, secreting too much insulin. By mid-morning, blood glucose crashes into reactive hypoglycaemia. At this moment, the sympathetic nervous system activates: cortisol and adrenaline surge. These stress hormones produce exactly the symptoms attributed to ADHD: inattention, hyperactivity, impulsivity, restlessness, emotional dysregulation, and difficulty following instructions. The consequences are immediate and observable in the classroom. Remove the reactive hypoglycaemia by eating a low-glycaemic breakfast instead, and these symptoms vanish within days. This is not coincidence; it is biochemistry.

Evidence Links Blood Sugar Dysregulation to ADHD Symptoms

Insulin resistance is common in children with ADHD

Multiple studies have demonstrated that children diagnosed with ADHD have significantly higher rates of insulin resistance, impaired glucose tolerance, and metabolic syndrome compared to neurotypical peers. A 2013 meta-analysis found that children with ADHD had consistently elevated fasting insulin levels and lower insulin sensitivity, even when body weight was controlled for. This is not random, it is mechanistic.

Dopamine dysregulation occurs in both true ADHD and sugar-dysregulated brains

ADHD is characterised by reduced dopamine signalling in the prefrontal cortex and striatum. Stimulant medications used to treat ADHD work by increasing dopamine availability. However, dopamine dysregulation also occurs in the context of chronic blood sugar dysregulation. As discussed in Chapter 1, the repeated cycling of glucose spikes and crashes leads to downregulation of dopamine D2 receptors, the same downregulation seen in true ADHD. A child caught in this metabolic cycle becomes progressively more inattentive, more impulsive, and more reward-seeking, appearing identical to a child with true neurodevelopmental ADHD.

Cognitive performance deteriorates within hours of high-glycaemic breakfasts

Controlled studies have shown that children consuming high-sugar breakfast foods show significantly poorer cognitive performance, sustained attention, and working memory compared to children consuming low-glycaemic breakfasts. These differences are evident within 2 to 3 hours of breakfast. In one study, children eating a high-sugar breakfast showed a 15 to 20 per cent decrement in attention and problem-solving ability within 2 hours, compared to children eating a low-glycaemic alternative. Repeat this pattern daily for years, and the cumulative impact on academic performance and self-esteem is severe.

The sugar-hyperactivity connection has a real metabolic basis

The popular belief that sugar makes children hyperactive has been largely dismissed by nutritionists, who argue that double-blind studies show no direct stimulant effect of sugar itself. However, this dismissal misses a critical point: sugar does not directly cause hyperactivity, but reactive hypoglycaemia does. The symptom profile is identical to ADHD because the underlying mechanism, sympathetic activation and cortisol/adrenaline release, is identical. Parents and teachers who observe a child becoming hyperactive and emotionally dysregulated after consuming sweets are accurately observing reactive hypoglycaemia, even if they lack the metabolic vocabulary to describe it.

The Critical Micronutrients for Developing Brains

Why deficiencies compound metabolic injury

Beyond blood sugar stability, the developing brain depends on a constellation of micronutrients that are systematically depleted in ultra-processed, high-sugar diets. Iron deficiency deserves special mention because it is one of the most common nutritional deficiencies in childhood, yet it is frequently overlooked in the evaluation of children with ADHD-like symptoms. Iron is a rate-limiting cofactor in dopamine synthesis, without adequate iron, the brain simply cannot produce sufficient dopamine. A child with iron deficiency anaemia presents with inattention, fatigue, poor academic performance, and reduced motivation, symptoms that are clinically indistinguishable from ADHD.

- **Zinc** supports neurotransmitter synthesis, insulin signalling, and synaptic plasticity. Deficiency presents as hyperactivity, irritability, impaired learning, and poor immunity.
- **Magnesium** regulates the NMDA receptor, modulates cortisol, and supports sleep and glucose metabolism. Deficiency produces anxiety, sleep problems, muscle tension, and ADHD-like symptoms.
- **Omega-3 fatty acids (DHA/EPA)** support myelination, neuronal membrane integrity, and synaptic plasticity. Deficiency manifests as poor attention, emotional dysregulation, and developmental delays.
- **B vitamins (B6, B12, folate)** are cofactors in neurotransmitter synthesis and myelin formation. Deficiency produces mood instability, irritability, brain fog, and poor concentration.
- **Vitamin D** supports neuroprotection and serotonin synthesis. Deficiency contributes to depression, poor immune function, and cognitive underperformance.

The Structural Tragedy of School Environments

How timing and available food create metabolic chaos

Here lies a structural tragedy: school canteens and vending machines in many countries continue to supply high-glycaemic, ultra-processed foods as the default option. But the timing is particularly damaging. Breakfast is served at 8:00 am, but core learning, numeracy, literacy, complex problem-solving, occurs between 9:00 am and 12:00 pm. If a child eats a high-sugar breakfast, the reactive hypoglycaemia window opens precisely during these critical learning hours. The child sits in a maths class struggling to focus, internally experiencing the sympathetic activation of reactive hypoglycaemia, branded as inattentive, diagnosed with ADHD, and placed on stimulants, when a low-glycaemic breakfast would have solved the problem entirely.

Evidence from schools that have implemented low-glycaemic breakfast and lunch programmes is striking. These programmes typically replace white bread with wholegrain alternatives, sugary cereals with oatmeal and eggs, sugary drinks with water and milk. Schools making these changes report improved cognitive performance, better behaviour, fewer classroom disruptions, and improved academic outcomes. The effect sizes are substantial, often 10 to 20 per cent improvements in test scores within weeks.

What parents can implement immediately

Protein-rich breakfasts prevent reactive hypoglycaemia. Eggs, Greek yoghurt, nut butters, and cheese eaten with whole-grain bread create stable, sustained glucose release. These breakfasts should contain 20 to 30 grams of protein. A breakfast of white toast and orange juice produces a glucose spike and crash; a breakfast of two eggs, whole-grain toast with almond butter, and a glass of milk produces stable glucose for 4 to 5 hours.

Eliminate sugary drinks entirely. Soft drinks, fruit juices, and flavoured milk drinks are liquid glucose bombs. A single 375 ml soft drink contains 40 grams of sugar, more than a child's recommended daily intake. Replace with water, unsweetened milk, or sparkling water. Reduce processed snack foods like crisps, biscuits, and granola bars. Replace with nuts, seeds, whole fruit, cheese, and hard-boiled eggs. Establish regular meal timing: children's brains require more frequent fuel than adults. A morning snack at 10:00 am (nuts, cheese, apple with almond butter) sustains glucose stability and maintains focus.

The Adolescent Perfect Storm: Screens, Sleep, and Blood Sugar

How three metabolic disruptors converge

Adolescents are experiencing a convergence of three metabolic disruptors simultaneously: screen use, sleep disruption, and high-sugar diet. Late-night screen use emits blue light that suppresses melatonin onset, delaying sleep by 30 to 90 minutes. This delay shortens the night, reducing deep non-REM sleep, the stage during which growth hormone is released and insulin sensitivity is highest. Simultaneously, screen use drives late-night snacking. The adolescent lies in bed scrolling through social media, compulsively eating high-sugar snacks while their melatonin is suppressed and their insulin sensitivity is at its nadir. The glucose spike occurs precisely when the body is least able to handle it.

The convergence is metabolically vicious. Poor sleep impairs insulin sensitivity. Late-night eating spikes glucose. Glucose spikes at night further impair insulin sensitivity. The adolescent wakes metabolically dysregulated, consumes another high-sugar breakfast, and the cycle perpetuates. The clinical manifestation is dramatic: adolescent depression, anxiety, and ADHD-like inattention have become epidemics precisely in parallel with the rise of smartphone use beginning around 2010–2012. The evidence suggests that metabolic dysregulation is a major contributing mechanism.

By establishing practical boundaries, you interrupt this cycle. Implement a screen curfew: no screens for at least one hour before bedtime. This allows melatonin to rise naturally. Keep the bedroom cool (65–68°F / 18–20°C), dark, and quiet. Finish eating at least three hours before bed. If hunger occurs in the evening, consume only protein and fat, foods that do not trigger glucose spikes. Get 15 to 30 minutes of sunlight exposure within one hour of waking to strengthen the circadian rhythm.

Supporting Children Naturally: The Metabolic Recovery Framework

The plate method adapted for children

At each meal, the child's plate should contain approximately half non-starchy vegetables (broccoli, carrots, spinach, peppers), one quarter lean protein (chicken, fish, eggs, legumes), and one quarter complex carbohydrates (sweet potato, wholegrain rice, oats). This ratio ensures adequate micronutrients, prevents reactive hypoglycaemia, and maintains satiety between meals. Children require eating every 3 to 4 hours to maintain stable glucose. A typical schedule might be: breakfast at 7:00 am, morning snack at 10:00 am, lunch at 12:30 pm, afternoon snack at 3:30 pm, dinner at 6:00 pm.

Reframing reward and emotional comfort

Many families use sweets, desserts, and high-sugar foods as rewards, punishment, or emotional comfort. A child learns that sugar equals love, sugar equals celebration, sugar equals comfort. This creates a powerful psychological-metabolic feedback loop that is extremely difficult to break. Instead, frame rewards around experiences (a trip to the park, extra time with a parent, a film night), physical activities, or genuinely nutritious foods made special. Homemade smoothie bowls, baked fruit with nuts, and cheese boards with fresh fruit become celebrations rather than processed sweets.

Physical activity as metabolic intervention

Exercise improves insulin sensitivity and dopamine signalling in developing brains. Children should engage in at least 60 minutes of moderate-intensity physical activity daily, a combination of aerobic activity and resistance training. Parents can normalise movement by exercising alongside their children, making family walks or bike rides part of the routine.

Identifying reactive hypoglycaemia through observation

When does your child have meltdowns? What did they eat 1 to 3 hours prior? If a child consistently has mood crashes, inattention, or aggressive outbursts at 10:30 am, and they ate a high-sugar breakfast at 8:00 am, reactive hypoglycaemia is the likely culprit. A single-blind dietary experiment, changing breakfast to low-glycaemic foods for one week, often produces undeniable evidence: the meltdowns and inattention disappear.

Key Takeaways

- Metabolic dysregulation in developing brains produces symptoms indistinguishable from ADHD; insulin resistance is common in children diagnosed with ADHD.
- Reactive hypoglycaemia creates inattention, hyperactivity, and emotional dysregulation through sympathetic nervous system activation, the same symptoms attributed to ADHD.
- Stable glucose depends on protein-rich, low-glycaemic breakfasts; regular meal timing (every 3–4 hours); and elimination of liquid sugars.
- Micronutrient deficiencies, particularly iron, zinc, magnesium, and B vitamins, compound metabolic injury and produce ADHD-like symptoms.
- Sleep disruption from late-night screens and poor sleep architecture impairs insulin sensitivity and perpetuates metabolic dysregulation in adolescents.

Next Steps

Understanding that your child's behavioural or emotional difficulties may have a metabolic root is empowering. It shifts the focus from psychiatric diagnosis and medication toward metabolic intervention, an approach that is evidence-based, accessible, and often produces rapid improvements. Reversing metabolic ADHD in a child requires compassion and patience, but the results are often dramatically rewarding. Parents often report that within one to two weeks of implementing metabolic changes, their child's behaviour transforms: meltdowns disappear, focus improves, mood stabilises, and academic performance rises.

The chapters that follow provide the detailed protocols, the specific foods to prioritise, the micronutrients to support, and the lifestyle practices that stabilise glucose and support nervous system regulation. By applying these principles in your child's daily life, you are not simply treating symptoms; you are supporting the foundational metabolic health from which a stable, resilient mind emerges.

References

Millichap, J. G., & Yee, M. M. (2012). The diet factor in attention-deficit/hyperactivity disorder. *Pediatrics*, 129(2), 330–337. https://doi.org/10.1542/peds.2011-3671

Ghanizadeh, A. (2012). Food and nutrient intake in children with attention deficit hyperactivity disorder. *Iranian Journal of Psychiatry*, 7(2), 89–93.

Wesnes, K. A., Pincock, C., Richardson, D., Helm, G., & Hails, R. (2003). Breakfast reduces declines in attention and memory over the morning in schoolchildren. *Appetite*, 41(3), 329–331. https://doi.org/10.1016/S0195-6663(03)00097-1

Richardson, A. J. (2006). Omega-3 fatty acids in ADHD and related neurodevelopmental disorders. *International Review of Psychiatry*, 18(2), 155–172. https://doi.org/10.1080/09540260600583031

Chapter 31: Your Micronutrient Toolkit – Building the Nutritional Foundation

The Nutrient Bankruptcy of Refined Foods

Introduction: Why micronutrients matter as much as macronutrients

Blood sugar dysregulation does not just starve the brain of energy, it depletes the micronutrients required to regulate that energy in the first place. The brain needs an intricate web of vitamins, minerals, and cofactors to convert glucose into usable energy, synthesise neurotransmitters, and maintain the structural integrity of neurons. This chapter consolidates all the supplementation evidence in one practical reference: what to take, why, in what doses and forms, and how to test rather than guess.

One of the most compelling bodies of evidence for micronutrient supplementation in mental health comes from the work of Professor Julia Rucklidge at the University of Canterbury. Rucklidge and colleagues have conducted a series of rigorous randomised controlled trials demonstrating that broad-spectrum micronutrient formulas, providing vitamins, minerals, and trace elements in physiological doses, can produce clinically significant improvements in mood, anxiety, stress, and ADHD symptoms. Her 2012 RCT conducted in the aftermath of the Christchurch earthquake found that adults receiving a broad-spectrum micronutrient formula reported significantly lower rates of anxiety, stress, and PTSD symptoms compared to controls, with a large effect size that persisted at follow-up. A subsequent trial published in the *British Journal of Psychiatry* found that adults with ADHD randomised to micronutrients showed significant improvements in inattention, emotional dysregulation, and overall functioning compared to placebo. Rucklidge's work is particularly important because it challenges the reductionist assumption that single-nutrient supplementation is sufficient, the brain, she argues, requires the full complement of micronutrients in synergistic combination.

This is why supplementation is not optional for those eating a modern diet, it is foundational. Each molecule of glucose burned for energy requires B vitamins as cofactors in the mitochondrial energy pathways. Each glucose spike triggers oxidative stress requiring magnesium, zinc, and selenium to activate antioxidant enzymes. Each blood sugar crash prompts a surge of cortisol requiring vitamin C and chromium for proper synthesis and regulation. Yet the ultra-processed foods delivering these excess calories are almost entirely devoid of these cofactors. The human body is left in a state of "nutrient theft", expending precious micronutrient reserves to process calories derived from foods that contain no micronutrients.

The Master Toolkit: Essential Nutrients and Their Roles

Magnesium: The stress-response regulator

Magnesium is your nervous system's most important mineral. It activates the insulin receptor, modulates the NMDA receptor (involved in anxiety and stress response), regulates cortisol, and supports sleep quality and mitochondrial ATP production. When magnesium is depleted, which is common in chronic stress and high-sugar diet, anxiety, insomnia, muscle cramps, restlessness, and blood sugar instability emerge. Therapeutic dose: 300–400 mg daily. Best form: Magnesium glycinate or malate for superior absorption and nervous system penetration. Food sources include dark leafy greens, pumpkin seeds, almonds, and dark chocolate (70%+).

Zinc: The dopamine and immunity co-factor

Zinc is required for insulin synthesis and secretion, testosterone production, dopamine modulation, and taste and smell. Deficiency presents as low mood, poor immunity, blood sugar swings, hair loss, and white spots on nails. Therapeutic dose: 15–30 mg daily. Best form: Picolinate or bisglycinate. Food sources: oysters, beef, pumpkin seeds, legumes, and cashews. Remember that high-dose zinc depletes copper, if supplementing above 30 mg daily, add 1–2 mg copper and monitor serum copper annually.

Chromium: The insulin sensitivity enhancer

Chromium enhances insulin receptor sensitivity, reduces carbohydrate cravings, and stabilises blood glucose. Deficiency produces intense carbohydrate cravings, blood sugar instability, and weight gain. Therapeutic dose: 200–400 mcg daily. Best form: Picolinate form (most bioavailable). Food sources: broccoli, beef, brewer's yeast, and whole grains. When taken 15 minutes before a carbohydrate-containing meal, chromium blunts the glucose spike by enhancing insulin sensitivity.

Thiamine (B1): The energy-production vitamin

Thiamine is essential for mitochondrial energy production, glucose metabolism, and the synthesis of acetylcholine and GABA. Deficiency produces fatigue, depression, anxiety, brain fog, and peripheral neuropathy. Therapeutic dose: 100–300 mg daily (benfotiamine preferred). Best form: Benfotiamine (fat-soluble, crosses the blood-brain barrier) or allithiamine. Food sources: pork, nutritional yeast, sunflower seeds, tahini, and brown rice.

B6 (Pyridoxine): The neurotransmitter builder

B6 is required for serotonin, dopamine, and GABA synthesis, homocysteine regulation, and immune function. Deficiency produces depression, anxiety, irritability, peripheral neuropathy, and skin issues. Therapeutic dose: 25–50 mg daily (P5P form preferred). Best form: Pyridoxal-5-phosphate (P5P) is the active form. Food sources: poultry, fish, chickpeas, bananas, avocados, and potatoes. Important caution: High-dose B6 (>200 mg daily long-term) can cause peripheral neuropathy, use the P5P form and keep doses moderate.

B12 (Cobalamin): The myelin and methylation co-factor

B12 is essential for myelin synthesis, methylation cycle function, neuronal energy production, homocysteine clearance, and DNA replication. Deficiency produces depression, cognitive decline, fatigue, and memory problems.

Therapeutic dose: 500–1000 mcg daily (oral) or 1000 mcg monthly (injection). Best form: Methylcobalamin (more active than cyanocobalamin). Food sources: meat, eggs, dairy, shellfish, and fortified nutritional yeast. Many people with psychiatric symptoms have "normal" total B12 but depleted holotranscobalamin (active B12), request this more specific test.

Folate (B9): The methylation and mood stabiliser

Folate is essential for DNA methylation, neurotransmitter synthesis, homocysteine regulation, and mood stability. Deficiency is strongly associated with depression, particularly SSRI-resistant depression, cognitive fog, and fatigue. Therapeutic dose: 400–800 mcg daily (dietary) or 1000–2000 mcg (therapeutic). Best form: Methylfolate (5-MTHF), especially if you carry MTHFR mutations. Approximately 30–40 per cent of the population carries at least one MTHFR mutation, impairing the conversion of folic acid to its active form, for these individuals, methylfolate is required for effectiveness. Food sources: leafy greens, legumes, asparagus, liver, and avocado.

Vitamin D3: The neuroprotection hormone

Vitamin D3 regulates insulin secretion and sensitivity, supports neuroprotection, modulates serotonin synthesis, and supports immune regulation. Deficiency contributes to depression, seasonal mood changes, immune dysfunction, and poor blood sugar control. Therapeutic dose (for deficiency correction): 2,000–5,000 IU daily; maintenance dose (for replete individuals): 1,000–2,000 IU daily. Higher end of range appropriate in winter or with limited sun exposure. Best form: D3 with K2 (K2 directs calcium to bones, not arteries). Food sources: sunlight exposure (15–30 minutes daily), oily fish, egg yolks, and sunlight-exposed mushrooms. Optimal range for mental health: 50–80 ng/mL (125–200 nmol/L).

Omega-3 (DHA/EPA): The neuroinflammation resolver

Omega-3 fatty acids support neuronal membrane integrity, anti-inflammatory signalling, BDNF support, and insulin sensitisation. Deficiency produces depression, anxiety, brain fog, dry skin, and inflammatory conditions. Therapeutic dose: 2–3 g EPA+DHA daily (therapeutic); 1–1.5 g for maintenance. Best form: Triglyceride-form fish oil (more bioavailable than ethyl ester). Food sources: oily fish (salmon, mackerel, sardines, herring), walnuts, flaxseed, and chia seeds.

Alpha Lipoic Acid (ALA): The mitochondrial antioxidant

Alpha Lipoic Acid is a mitochondrial antioxidant that improves insulin sensitivity, reduces advanced glycation end-products (AGEs), and can reverse neuropathy. Therapeutic dose: 300–600 mg daily (higher for neuropathy: 1200 mg daily in divided doses). Best form: R-ALA (right-handed form; S-ALA is less effective). Food sources: spinach, broccoli, organ meats, tomato, and Brussels sprouts.

Berberine: The AMPK activator

Berberine activates AMPK, enabling insulin-independent glucose uptake, and has blood sugar regulation efficacy comparable to metformin. Therapeutic dose: 500 mg 2–3 times daily with meals. Best form: Standardised extract (minimum 97% berberine). Important: Berberine is metabolised by cytochrome P450 enzymes in the liver and may interact with medications, consult a pharmacist before combining with statins, blood pressure medications, immunosuppressants, or some psychiatric medications.

Vitamin C (Ascorbate): The cortisol regulator

Vitamin C is an antioxidant that supports cortisol modulation, collagen synthesis, and counters glucose-ascorbate antagonism. Deficiency produces fatigue, poor wound healing, low immune function, and easy bruising. Therapeutic dose: 500–1000 mg daily. Best form: Buffered ascorbate (gentler on the gastrointestinal tract than ascorbic acid). Food sources: citrus fruits, kiwi, capsicum, broccoli, and strawberries.

Testing Before Supplementing: The Intelligence-First Approach

Why guessing is inefficient and potentially harmful

The most common mistake people make with supplementation is treating it as guesswork. They read about magnesium, assume they might be deficient, take high-dose supplements, and hope for improvement. This is inefficient and can be counterproductive. Testing before supplementing gives you metabolic literacy, you know your actual status rather than guessing.

The gold standard tests

Red blood cell (RBC) magnesium is more accurate than serum magnesium because only 1 per cent of body magnesium is in the serum, the rest is intracellular. Serum magnesium can appear "normal" while intracellular magnesium is severely depleted. Reference range: 5.0–6.5 mg/dL (RBC magnesium). Values below 5.0 mg/dL indicate deficiency.

Serum zinc and copper should always be checked together, zinc depletes copper at high supplemental doses, and copper excess impairs zinc absorption. Serum zinc reference: 60–120 mcg/dL (fasting). A zinc-to-copper ratio below 8:1 suggests zinc deficiency; above 12:1 suggests zinc excess and possible copper depletion.

25-hydroxy vitamin D (25-OH Vitamin D) is the best indicator of vitamin D status. Optimal range for mental health and bone health: 50–80 ng/mL (125–200 nmol/L). Many "normal" ranges extend down to 30 ng/mL, but mental health outcomes improve markedly above 50 ng/mL.

Serum B12 and active B12 (holotranscobalamin) provide the most accurate picture. Standard serum B12 can be misleading because it includes both active B12 and inactive analogues. Reference ranges: Total B12 200–900 pg/mL (serum); Holotranscobalamin >35 pmol/L (optimal >100 pmol/L for mental health).

Serum folate and MTHFR genetic status work together. Serum folate reference: >5.4 ng/mL. However, genetic testing for MTHFR variants determines whether you metabolise folic acid efficiently or require methylfolate supplementation. Approximately 30–40 per cent of the population carries at least one MTHFR mutation.

Fasting insulin and HOMA-IR (Homeostatic Model Assessment for Insulin Resistance) comprise arguably the single most important metabolic test, yet it is ordered by fewer than 10 per cent of general practitioners. Fasting glucose can be normal while fasting insulin is elevated, a sign of early-stage insulin resistance. Fasting insulin reference: optimal <5 mIU/L; borderline 5–10 mIU/L; significant insulin resistance >10 mIU/L.

Synergistic Stacking: Pairing Nutrients for Maximum Effect

Pairs that amplify each other

Magnesium and B6 (as P5P) are both required for the synthesis of serotonin, dopamine, and GABA. Magnesium activates the enzymes that convert B6 to its active form. When taken together, they amplify each other's neurological effects. Typical pairing: 300 mg magnesium glycinate + 30 mg P5P.

Vitamin D3 and K2 work synergistically. Vitamin D increases intestinal absorption of calcium, but without adequate K2, calcium deposits in arteries rather than bones. K2 directs calcium into skeleton and teeth and away from soft tissue. Take together: 2000–5000 IU D3 + 100–200 mcg K2 (MK-7 form is most bioavailable).

Zinc and B6 (as P5P) both support immune function and mood. They work synergistically for neurological resilience.

Omega-3 and Vitamin E pair well because omega-3 fatty acids are prone to oxidation. Vitamin E is a fat-soluble antioxidant that protects omega-3 from oxidative damage. Most quality fish oil supplements include vitamin E for this reason.

Critical separations to prevent interference

Zinc and iron should be taken separately because both compete for absorption via divalent metal transporters. If you need both supplements, take zinc in the morning with coffee (which reduces iron absorption) and iron in the evening with vitamin C (which enhances iron absorption). Separate by at least 2 hours.

Calcium and magnesium should be taken at different meals because both compete for absorption. Take one at breakfast and one at dinner, separated by at least 6 hours.

Iron and coffee/tea should be separated because the polyphenols in coffee and tea strongly inhibit iron absorption. If taking supplemental iron, avoid coffee/tea for at least one hour before and two hours after the supplement.

Timing and Implementation: The Practical Protocol

Morning protocol (upon waking or with breakfast)

B vitamins (B1, B6, B12, folate) are energising and should be taken early in the day to avoid interfering with sleep. Vitamin D3 with K2 requires dietary fat for absorption, so take with a meal containing fat. Omega-3 is better tolerated with food and the fat content enhances absorption.

With meals (breakfast, lunch)

Chromium picolinate, taken 15 minutes before eating a carbohydrate-containing meal, blunts the glucose spike by enhancing insulin sensitivity. Berberine is taken with the largest carbohydrate-containing meal of the day to maximise blood sugar stabilisation. Alpha Lipoic Acid is taken with food to enhance absorption and reduce gastrointestinal upset. Zinc is taken with food to avoid nausea and reduce absorption interference.

Evening protocol (1–2 hours before bed)

Magnesium glycinate 300–400 mg taken 30–60 minutes before bed promotes sleep quality and stabilises blood glucose overnight. The liver's endogenous glucose production is enhanced by magnesium, supporting stable blood glucose while sleeping. Vitamin C (buffered ascorbate) if stressed or ill supports adrenal function and immune recovery during sleep.

Flexible timing (morning or evening, but consistent)

Thiamine/Benfotiamine should be taken consistently with breakfast to support daytime energy production. The timing is less critical than consistency.

The Food-First Philosophy

Supplements are tools for correcting deficiencies created by modern diets and modern life, limited sun exposure, processed foods, chronic stress. They do not replace the synergistic matrix of nutrients found in whole foods. A high-quality diet containing abundant vegetables, fatty fish, eggs, nuts, seeds, and legumes will provide most micronutrients in forms and ratios optimised by millennia of human nutrition. Supplements fill specific gaps; they do not substitute for genuine food. The combination of targeted testing and strategic supplementation is how you move from guessing to knowing, and from managing symptoms to genuine metabolic restoration.

Key Takeaways

- Refined sugar metabolism aggressively consumes micronutrients; supplementation addresses specific deficiencies created by modern diets and chronic stress.
- Testing before supplementing (red blood cell magnesium, serum zinc, 25-OH vitamin D, active B12, MTHFR status) provides intelligence rather than guesswork.
- Synergistic pairs amplify effectiveness: magnesium + B6, vitamin D3 + K2, zinc + B6, omega-3 + vitamin E.
- Critical separations prevent interference: zinc and iron at different times, calcium and magnesium at different meals, iron away from coffee/tea.
- Timing matters: B vitamins in morning, magnesium in evening, zinc with meals, chromium before carbohydrates.

Next Steps

By consolidating supplementation into a practical toolkit, you gain the ability to address specific metabolic deficiencies with precision rather than spray-and-pray approaches. The chapters that follow show how these micronutrients work within the broader framework of metabolic psychiatry, supporting sleep, regulating stress hormones, stabilising mood, and enabling the brain's own healing processes. Begin with testing. Identify your specific deficiencies. Then supplement strategically, timing your intake for maximum absorption and effect. This intelligence-first approach transforms supplementation from a peripheral wellness activity into a central pillar of metabolic restoration.

References

Rucklidge, J. J., Andridge, R., Gorman, B., Blampied, N., Gordon, H., & Boggis, A. (2012). Shaken but unstirred? Effects of micronutrients on stress and trauma after an earthquake: RCT evidence comparing formulas and doses. *Human Psychopharmacology: Clinical and Experimental*, 27(5), 440–454. https://doi.org/10.1002/hup.2246

Rucklidge, J. J., Frampton, C. M., Gorman, B., & Boggis, A. (2014). Vitamin-mineral treatment of attention-deficit hyperactivity disorder in adults: Double-blind randomised placebo-controlled trial. *British Journal of Psychiatry*, 204(4), 306–315. https://doi.org/10.1192/bjp.bp.113.132126

Rucklidge, J. J., & Kaplan, B. J. (2016). Nutrition and mental health. *Clinical Psychological Science*, 4(6), 1082–1084. https://doi.org/10.1177/2167702616641050

Razzaque, M. S. (2018). The dualistic role of vitamin D in vascular calcification. *Nutrients*, 10(5), 652. https://doi.org/10.3390/nu10050652

Mohammadpour, N., Jazayeri, S., Tehrani-Doost, M., Djalali, M., Hosseini, M., Effatpanah, M., Davari-Ashtiani, R., & Karami, E. (2018). Effect of vitamin D supplementation as adjunctive therapy to methylphenidate on ADHD symptoms: A randomised, double blind, placebo-controlled trial. *Nutritional Neuroscience*, 21(3), 202–209. https://doi.org/10.1080/1028415X.2016.1262097

Richardson, A. J. (2006). Omega-3 fatty acids in ADHD and related neurodevelopmental disorders. *International Review of Psychiatry*, 18(2), 155–172. https://doi.org/10.1080/09540260600583031

Millichap, J. G., & Yee, M. M. (2012). The diet factor in attention-deficit/hyperactivity disorder. *Pediatrics*, 129(2), 330–337. https://doi.org/10.1542/peds.2011-3671

Chapter 32: Trauma, Cortisol, and Metabolic Dysregulation – The Hidden Link

When the Past Lives in the Body

Introduction: Trauma physiology and metabolic dysfunction are deeply entangled

Trauma does not exist only in memory. It lives in the body, inscribed into the nervous system, encoded in hormonal feedback loops, embedded in how your brain and body respond to perceived threat. The person with treatment-resistant depression may not primarily need more serotonin. They may need cortisol regulation. The individual with PTSD-driven hyperarousal may be kept physiologically activated, in part, by elevated blood glucose. Trauma physiology and metabolic dysfunction are deeply entangled, and treating one without understanding the other leaves both incompletely addressed.

Understanding this trauma-metabolism connection transforms how we approach healing. It means that supporting metabolic stability becomes an act of nervous system repair. It means that healing the body genuinely supports healing the mind, and vice versa. Metabolic psychiatry is not peripheral to trauma recovery, it is central to it.

The HPA Axis: From Protective Response to Chronic Dysregulation

The three-tiered stress system and its normal function

The hypothalamic-pituitary-adrenal axis is a three-tiered communication system that orchestrates the body's response to perceived threat. Under acute stress, a near-miss car accident, a confrontation, the response is deeply adaptive. Your hypothalamus releases corticotropin-releasing hormone (CRH), which stimulates your pituitary to release adrenocorticotropic hormone (ACTH), which in turn triggers your adrenal glands to release cortisol. Cortisol is a glucocorticoid. Its metabolic effects are rapid and purposeful: it promotes hepatic gluconeogenesis (the synthesis of glucose from non-carbohydrate sources), enhances glycogenolysis (the breakdown of stored glycogen), suppresses insulin secretion, and increases circulating glucose. In the ancestral context, this was brilliant. Your body needed to raise blood glucose to fuel the muscles required for fight or flight.

But trauma changes this equation. In individuals who have experienced childhood adverse events, significant life trauma, or are living with post-traumatic stress disorder, the HPA axis becomes chronically dysregulated, trapping the body in one of two pathological patterns. This dysregulation is not a psychological phenomenon, it is encoded in the body's neurochemistry and metabolic function.

Pattern One: HPA axis hyperreactivity

In many trauma survivors, and in a substantial proportion of individuals with depression and anxiety, the HPA axis becomes hyperactive. Cortisol remains chronically elevated, or spikes exaggerated in response to minor stressors. This perpetuates the metabolic state of threat: blood glucose remains chronically elevated, insulin secretion remains high in an attempt to manage the glucose, and the body accumulates visceral (abdominal) fat. The research is unambiguous: individuals with histories of trauma have higher baseline cortisol levels, flatter cortisol curves across the day, and exaggerated cortisol reactivity to stress. This hyperreactivity predicts metabolic syndrome, diabetes, cardiovascular disease, and depression. The body has learned that threat is ubiquitous, and it maintains metabolic vigilance accordingly.

Pattern Two: HPA axis blunting

A smaller subset of trauma survivors develop the opposite pattern: a blunted or flattened HPA axis, where cortisol fails to rise appropriately in response to stress. This hypocortisolism is particularly common in individuals with chronic PTSD characterised by numbing, avoidance, and emotional dissociation. Paradoxically, this flat cortisol curve is not protective, it leaves the body unable to mount an appropriate physiological response to real threats. The result is extreme fatigue, profound inflammatory hypersensitivity (because cortisol normally provides immunosuppressive braking on inflammation), heightened pain sensitivity, and often a sense of complete energetic collapse. This pattern is seen in fibromyalgia and myalgic encephalomyelitis/chronic fatigue syndrome, which frequently co-occur with this hypocortisolism pattern.

The ACE Study: How Early Adversity Becomes Metabolic Disease Decades Later

The landmark findings

In 1998, Vincent Felitti and colleagues published a landmark epidemiological study linking childhood adverse experiences (ACEs), including physical, emotional, and sexual abuse; parental separation; parental substance misuse; and parental mental illness, to chronic disease outcomes in adulthood. The study followed over 17,000 adults, linking their ACE scores to their health outcomes decades later. The findings were striking and unambiguous: individuals with four or more ACEs had dramatically elevated rates of diabetes (4.6-fold increased risk), metabolic syndrome (3.0-fold increase), depression (4.5-fold increase), and anxiety disorders (3.5-fold increase). These were not modest associations, they were large, robust, and dose-dependent. The more adversity an individual had experienced in childhood, the greater the metabolic disease burden in adulthood.

The mechanism: Nervous system learning

The mechanism is clear: early trauma dysregulates the developing HPA axis during a critical window when the stress-response system is being wired. The nervous system learns, put simply, that threat is ubiquitous and persistent. This learned hypervigilance becomes embedded in the brain's architecture, maintaining a chronic state of metabolic activation, elevated cortisol, elevated glucose, suppressed insulin sensitivity, for decades. What is striking is that the metabolic consequences of early trauma play out silently for years. A 40-year-old woman with an ACE score of 5 may not show obvious psychiatric symptoms, yet her fasting glucose may already be elevated, her visceral fat may be accumulating, her insulin resistance may be developing, all driven by a dysregulated HPA axis responding to threats that are no longer present. This is why metabolic psychiatry's focus on blood sugar stability is not just psychiatric treatment; it is an act of trauma recovery.

Cortisol, Insulin Resistance, and Visceral Fat: The Metabolic Cascade

How chronic cortisol drives metabolic dysfunction

When cortisol remains chronically elevated, the liver is continuously stimulated to produce glucose via gluconeogenesis. This drives persistent mild hyperglycaemia, not severe enough to meet diagnostic criteria for diabetes, but enough to be pathological. The pancreas responds by secreting more insulin, attempting to lower the circulating glucose. Over months and years, as this pattern persists, the body's cells become less responsive to insulin's signal, they develop insulin resistance. Paradoxically, the compensatory hyperinsulinemia worsens the metabolic dysfunction: high insulin levels suppress lipolysis (fat breakdown), promote de novo lipogenesis (fat synthesis), and drive fat storage rather than fat utilisation.

But cortisol's metabolic effects extend beyond glucose. Cortisol selectively promotes visceral (abdominal or omental) fat deposition through multiple mechanisms: cortisol increases the density of glucocorticoid receptors in visceral adipose tissue, making these fat cells highly sensitive to cortisol's lipogenic signals. Visceral fat is not metabolically inert, it is highly active, secreting inflammatory cytokines including tumour necrosis factor-alpha (TNF-α), interleukin-6 (IL-6), and resistin. These cytokines circulate systemically and to the brain, where they amplify neuroinflammation and directly impair insulin signalling in key metabolic centres including the hypothalamus and hippocampus.

The vicious cycle

This creates a vicious feedback loop: trauma dysregulates the HPA axis → chronic cortisol elevation → hepatic glucose overproduction and visceral fat accumulation → visceral adipose tissue-derived inflammation → worsening insulin resistance in the brain and periphery → further HPA axis reactivity → perpetuation of the cycle. Breaking this loop requires intervention at multiple points simultaneously: normalising cortisol through nervous system regulation, stabilising blood glucose through dietary choices, reducing visceral fat through metabolic intervention, and addressing the inflammatory burden through both nutrition and movement.

The Gut-Trauma Axis: How Dysbiosis Perpetuates Metabolic Dysregulation

Stress hormones reshape the microbiota

The gut microbiome, that ecosystem of trillions of microorganisms living in your intestinal tract, is highly sensitive to stress and trauma. Stress hormones including cortisol and catecholamines alter gut motility, increase permeability, and change the secretion patterns of antimicrobial peptides. The sympathetic nervous system (activated during fight-or-flight) directly suppresses secretion of immunoglobulin A and mucus, both of which protect the intestinal lining. Over time, this chronic stress-driven suppression of protective barriers permits increased intestinal permeability, the phenomenon colloquially known as "leaky gut", which allows bacterial lipopolysaccharides and other microbial antigens to cross the intestinal epithelium and enter the bloodstream, triggering systemic immune activation.

Critically, stress hormones also reshape the microbiota itself. Cortisol and catecholamines selectively suppress the growth of short-chain fatty acid (SCFA)-producing bacteria, particularly species of Faecalibacterium, Roseburia, and other Firmicutes, while favouring the growth of pathogenic species. This shift in microbial composition directly impairs glucose metabolism: the loss of SCFA-producing bacteria means less butyrate production, and butyrate is a critical signalling molecule that improves insulin sensitivity at both the intestinal and systemic level. Without adequate SCFA production, the intestinal barrier weakens further, and metabolic dysregulation accelerates.

Bidirectional communication through the vagus nerve

The gut communicates directly with the brain via the vagus nerve, the longest cranial nerve, which carries afferent (brain-ward) signals from the gut that inform the brain about metabolic and immune status. A dysbiotic microbiota, depleted of SCFA producers, sends signals of metabolic distress up the vagus nerve, perpetuating the brain's interpretation of threat and maintaining HPA axis activation. This bidirectional communication is why microbiome restoration is not a peripheral intervention in trauma recovery; it is central to nervous system healing. Evidence supports this mechanism: individuals with high ACE scores show altered microbiome composition compared to those with low ACE scores, characterised by reduced abundance of Lactobacillus and Bifidobacterium species, key SCFA producers and promoters of intestinal barrier integrity.

Nervous System Regulation: How Vagal Tone Directly Improves Metabolic Health

The bidirectional link between vagal tone and insulin sensitivity

One of the most under-appreciated connections in medicine links parasympathetic nervous system tone, specifically, vagal tone, directly to insulin sensitivity. This connection is bidirectional and powerful. The vagus nerve is the longest cranial nerve, carrying parasympathetic (rest-and-digest) signals throughout the body. High vagal tone, a marker of a relaxed, well-regulated nervous system, directly promotes insulin-stimulated glucose uptake in skeletal muscle and suppresses hepatic glucose production. Conversely, low vagal tone, reflecting chronic sympathetic dominance (the fight-or-flight state), impairs insulin signalling and promotes persistently elevated blood glucose.

The mechanism involves the vagus nerve's direct innervation of the pancreatic islets: high vagal tone stimulates acetylcholine release, which amplifies insulin secretion from beta cells and promotes alpha cell suppression (reducing glucagon). Simultaneously, vagal activation promotes insulin sensitivity in peripheral tissues through cholinergic signalling pathways. This means that nervous system healing is metabolic healing. A person with a history of trauma who develops the capacity to regulate their nervous system, to shift from hypervigilance to a state of relative safety and calm, simultaneously becomes more insulin-sensitive and metabolically efficient.

Practical techniques for vagal activation

Slow diaphragmatic breathing techniques such as 4-7-8 breathing (inhale for 4 counts, hold for 7, exhale for 8) and resonance breathing (approximately 6 breaths per minute, often achieved through guided breathing apps) acutely shift autonomic balance toward the parasympathetic. Even brief periods of slow breathing,5 to 10 minutes, reduce cortisol, lower blood glucose, and improve insulin sensitivity acutely. Regular practice (10 to 20 minutes daily) produces sustained improvements in HPA axis regulation and metabolic markers.

Graduated cold exposure, starting with short cold showers (15 to 30 seconds of cold water at the end of a warm shower) and progressing to longer exposure, activates the vagus nerve and recalibrates noradrenergic regulation. Cold exposure also stimulates the sympathetic nervous system acutely, which might seem counterintuitive, but repeated controlled cold exposure actually reduces baseline sympathetic tone and improves parasympathetic capacity. The metabolic benefits include improved insulin sensitivity and enhanced thermogenic capacity.

Slow, deliberate movement practices, particularly those emphasising breath-to-movement synchronisation, directly activate the vagus nerve through vagal afferents responding to postural changes. Hatha yoga, Yin yoga, and somatic-focused movement practices produce measurable improvements in vagal tone (as assessed by heart rate variability) and corresponding improvements in insulin sensitivity and stress hormone regulation.

Safe relational connection activates what Stephen Porges calls the ventral vagus, the social engagement pathway. Safety signals received from trusted relationships, eye contact, vocal prosody, attuned presence, activate the ventral vagus, creating a physiological state of safety that simultaneously reduces HPA axis reactivity and improves metabolic efficiency. This is why trauma-informed, relational therapeutic approaches are not luxuries; they are metabolic necessities.

A Comprehensive Metabolic Recovery Framework for Trauma Survivors

Recognition and metabolic compassion

Begin with the understanding that your body's dysregulated stress response, whether hyperreactive or blunted, is not a character flaw. It is an adaptive response that protected you when threats were real. Healing involves gradually retraining your nervous system to distinguish genuine present-moment danger from echoes of past trauma. This retraining requires both psychological work and metabolic support.

Blood sugar stability as the foundation

Stable blood glucose is foundational to nervous system regulation. Hypoglycaemic episodes, drops in blood glucose, are detected by the body as threats, triggering adrenaline release, HPA axis activation, and symptoms of anxiety or panic. For trauma survivors, whose threat-detection systems are already sensitised, this glucose-driven "false alarm" can retrigger trauma responses. Ensuring three regular, balanced meals (protein + fat + fibre-rich carbohydrate) prevents these glucose crashes and removes a source of iatrogenic HPA activation.

Targeted supplementation for HPA normalisation

Several evidence-based supplements support HPA axis regulation. Magnesium glycinate (300 to 400 mg daily, preferably in the evening) directly modulates the HPA axis; magnesium deficiency amplifies cortisol reactivity. Glycine additionally supports GABA synthesis and has its own anxiolytic properties. B-complex vitamins (preferably methylated forms) support the synthesis of both serotonin and GABA, which require adequate B vitamins, particularly B6, B12, and folate. Trauma survivors often have depleted B vitamin status due to chronic stress. Ashwagandha (KSM-66 extract) has strong evidence for cortisol normalisation, both reducing elevated cortisol in those with hyperactivity and supporting cortisol in those with blunting. Dosing: 300 to 500 mg daily in divided doses. Omega-3 polyunsaturated fatty acids (2 to 3 grams daily of combined EPA and DHA) support neuroinflammation resolution and improve HPA axis regulation.

Gentle, progressive movement

Exercise supports trauma recovery, but the type of exercise matters. High-intensity exercise, while beneficial for many, can retrigger trauma responses in some individuals due to the sympathetic activation and physical stress. Begin with gentle, mindful movement: walking in nature (which additionally provides the nervous system-regulating benefits of green space), yoga, tai chi, or swimming. Progress to moderate-intensity aerobic exercise and resistance training only as the nervous system demonstrates capacity. The goal is to gradually expand the window of tolerance, the range of intensities and stressors the nervous system can process without dysregulation.

Professional support as integration

Metabolic psychiatry works alongside, not instead of, trauma-informed therapy. The most effective approaches integrate somatic therapy (which works directly with the body's stress responses), cognitive-behavioural therapy or EMDR (for processing traumatic memories), and metabolic support. If medication is indicated, work with a clinician familiar with both psychopharmacology and nutritional psychiatry to optimise the combination.

Key Takeaways

- Trauma dysregulates the HPA axis, creating either chronic cortisol elevation (hyperreactivity) or cortisol blunting (hypocortisolism), both of which impair metabolic function and mental health.
- Chronic cortisol elevation drives hepatic glucose overproduction, visceral fat accumulation, and systemic inflammation, creating metabolic syndrome through a physiological cascade that began with trauma.
- The gut microbiome is dysregulated by trauma; SCFA-producing bacteria are depleted, weakening the intestinal barrier and amplifying neuroinflammation through the gut-brain axis.
- High vagal tone, achieved through slow breathing, cold exposure, movement practices, and safe relational connection, directly improves insulin sensitivity and reduces HPA axis reactivity.
- Trauma recovery is metabolic recovery: stable blood glucose, targeted supplementation, and nervous system regulation work together to heal the dysregulated stress response.

Next Steps

Understanding that your trauma physiology has a metabolic dimension is deeply empowering. It means that supporting your metabolic health, eating regular, balanced meals; supplementing strategically; practising nervous system regulation techniques, is not peripheral to healing from trauma; it is central. The body's dysregulated stress response can be retrained, and this retraining is facilitated by metabolic stability and nervous system healing practices. As you implement the interventions described in this chapter, stable blood glucose, targeted supplementation, and vagal activation techniques, you are not merely managing psychiatric symptoms; you are gradually recalibrating the nervous system's threat-detection system, teaching your body that safety is possible. This is the path from trauma's grip toward genuine resilience and healing.

References

Danese, A., & McEwen, B. S. (2012). Adverse childhood experiences, allostasis, allostatic load, and age-related disease. *Physiology & Behavior*, 106(1), 29–39. https://doi.org/10.1016/j.physbeh.2011.08.011

Felitti, V. J., Anda, R. F., Nordenberg, D., Williamson, D. F., Spitz, A. M., Edwards, V., ... & Marks, J. S. (1998). Relationship of childhood abuse and household dysfunction to many of the leading causes of death in adults: The Adverse Childhood Experiences (ACE) Study. *American Journal of Preventive Medicine*, 14(4), 245–258. https://doi.org/10.1016/S0749-3797(98)00017-8

McEwen, B. S. (2007). Physiology and neurobiology of stress and adaptation: Central role of the brain. *Physiological Reviews*, 87(3), 873–904. https://doi.org/10.1152/physrev.00041.2006

Hemmings, S. M. J., Malan-Müller, S., van den Heuvel, L. L., Demmitt, B. A., Stanislawski, M. A., Smith, D. G., ... & Seedat, S. (2017). The microbiome in posttraumatic stress disorder and trauma-exposed controls: An exploratory study. *Psychosomatic Medicine*, 79(8), 936–946. https://doi.org/10.1097/PSY.0000000000000512

Porges, S. W. (2001). The polyvagal theory: Phylogenetic substrates of a social nervous system. *International Journal of Psychophysiology*, 42(2), 123–146. https://doi.org/10.1016/S0167-8760(01)00162-3

Chapter 33: Your 8-Week Action Plan – From Knowledge to Implementation

---

Where Science Becomes Your Life

Introduction: Translating research into lived metabolic recovery

Knowing the science is not the same as knowing what to do on Monday morning. By this point in the book, you understand why blood sugar stability matters, how gut health and inflammation influence mood, how nutrient deficiencies drive psychiatric symptoms, and how trauma and metabolic dysfunction reinforce each other. What remains is the question every reader is asking: where do I actually start? This chapter answers it with a concrete, week-by-week protocol, grounded in the evidence, sequenced for real life, and designed for the version of yourself who is tired, uncertain, and beginning anyway.

This chapter is your practical roadmap, an 8-week protocol designed to systematically address the blood sugar foundations of mental health, building layer by layer from the ground up. It is not a rigid prescription. It is not a diet that demands perfection. It is a flexible framework designed for real people, living real lives, with real constraints. The goal is progress, not perfection. Begin where you are. Use what you have. Do what you can.

Your Starting Point: The Baseline Assessment

Before you begin any metabolic intervention, take a baseline. This serves two essential purposes: it identifies significant deficiencies or dysregulations that require attention, and it provides a concrete benchmark against which you can measure progress. These tests are not luxuries, they are information, and information is power.

The tests that matter most include fasting glucose (screens for insulin resistance; reference: 3.9–5.5 mmol/L), fasting insulin plus HOMA-IR (the most sensitive early marker; fasting insulin optimal <5 mIU/L, borderline 5–10 mIU/L, elevated >10 mIU/L; HOMA-IR <2.0), HbA1c (reflects 3-month average glucose; reference: <5.7%), vitamin D (deficiency impairs mood and insulin secretion; optimal 50–80 ng/mL), full blood count plus ferritin (identifies iron deficiency; ferritin >50 µg/L), serum B12 and folate (critical for neurotransmitter synthesis; B12 >400 pg/mL), magnesium (red blood cell magnesium is more accurate than serum; >5.0 mg/dL), and thyroid panel (TSH 1–2.5 mIU/L, with free T3 and T4 in upper range). Where possible, obtain these through your GP, as they are typically funded by the NHS. If your GP is reluctant, seek a private laboratory or a nutritionist who can order them.

Weeks 1–2: Stabilise the Foundation

Remove the most metabolically disruptive foods

In these first two weeks, focus on removing the most metabolically disruptive foods, not because you are "bad" for eating them, but because their effects on your blood glucose and mood are so immediate and so damaging that removing them creates rapid, noticeable improvement.

Eliminate liquid sugars: soft drinks, energy drinks, and fruit juices (even freshly squeezed versions spike glucose as dramatically as soft drinks). Discontinue sweetened coffee drinks (lattes with syrup, sugary tea). Eliminate breakfast foods high in refined carbohydrates: sugary cereals, pastries, white bread, muffins, pancakes with syrup. These foods create the metabolic chaos described throughout this book, rapid glucose spikes followed by crashes that trigger afternoon anxiety, irritability, and intense sugar cravings.

Replace with a protein + fat breakfast within one hour of waking. This is non-negotiable. Examples include three whole eggs with vegetables and butter or olive oil; Greek yoghurt with nuts and berries; nut butter on sourdough (if tolerated) or on oatmeal; smoked salmon with avocado and cucumber. The protein and fat slow glucose absorption, stabilise insulin, and dramatically improve mood and cognitive function throughout the morning. You will notice this improvement within days.

Establish consistent meal timing and sleep

Begin eating at consistent times, three meals per day, no more than 4–5 hours apart. This consistency trains your metabolic and circadian systems, improving insulin sensitivity and normalising hunger and satiety signals. Establish a fixed wake time (within 30 minutes every day, including weekends) and a consistent bedtime. This synchronises your circadian rhythm, improving cortisol regulation, insulin sensitivity, and mood. Begin dimming lights at 9 PM. Remove screens from the bedroom; blue light suppresses melatonin. Aim for 7–9 hours of sleep nightly.

Your first supplement: Magnesium

Magnesium glycinate, 300 mg taken with dinner or before bed, is your HPA axis down-regulator and sleep enhancer. Avoid magnesium oxide (which causes diarrhoea); glycinate is well-absorbed and has its own anxiolytic effects.

By the end of Week 2, you should notice: improved energy in the morning, fewer afternoon energy crashes, reduced sugar cravings, better sleep, and improved mood stability. These changes occur because you have stabilised the blood glucose swings that were driving neuroinflammation and dysregulating your nervous system. This is your proof of concept, evidence that the metabolic approach works.

Weeks 3–4: Build the Plate

Introduce structural changes to meal composition

Now that the foundation is stable, introduce structural changes to how you construct meals. These changes embed the macronutrient principles discussed throughout this book into a simple, sustainable framework. At lunch and dinner, divide your plate into three sections: 50 per cent non-starchy vegetables (leafy greens, broccoli, cauliflower, carrots, peppers, courgettes, mushrooms, tomatoes), 25 per cent protein (chicken, fish, eggs, legumes, tofu), and 25 per cent complex carbohydrates (sweet potato, brown rice, quinoa, oats). This simple visual framework ensures that every meal contains adequate fibre, adequate protein, and adequate non-processed carbohydrate.

Fibre at every meal and macronutrient sequencing

Vegetables, legumes, and whole grains contain both insoluble fibre (which provides bulk and supports bowel regularity) and soluble fibre (which is fermented by the microbiome to produce short-chain fatty acids). Fibre is a metabolic magic bullet: it slows glucose absorption, feeds beneficial bacteria, improves insulin sensitivity, and supports stable mood. Aim for at least 25 grams of fibre daily (ideally 30–40 grams), distributed across meals. At each meal, eat vegetables and protein before you eat carbohydrates. This simple sequencing reduces the postprandial glucose spike by approximately 30–35 per cent, as measured by continuous glucose monitoring.

Postprandial glucose blunting and supplementation

Immediately after lunch and dinner, take a 10-minute walk, even a slow walk around your home or garden. Muscle contraction increases glucose uptake independently of insulin, directly blunting the postprandial glucose spike. This is not exercise; it is a metabolic hack that requires minimal time and produces remarkable results.

Introduce supplementation: Vitamin D3 (2,000–3,000 IU daily with breakfast) supports mood, insulin secretion, and immune function. Omega-3 fish oil or algal omega-3 (2 grams daily of combined EPA and DHA) reduces neuroinflammation and supports mood stability.

By the end of Week 4, your blood glucose swings should be substantially smaller, and your mood should be more stable. You are learning to construct meals that support your mental health. This is the beginning of food literacy, understanding that food is information, and that what you eat directly shapes how you feel.

Weeks 5–6: Deepen the Protocol

Time-restricted eating and microbiome restoration

These weeks focus on deeper metabolic optimisation and microbiome restoration. Consider introducing a 12-hour eating window, for example, eating between 8 AM and 8 PM, with a 12-hour fasting window from 8 PM to 8 AM. This is the gentlest form of time-restricted eating, and it has multiple metabolic benefits: it improves insulin sensitivity, reduces visceral fat accumulation, enhances autophagy (cellular cleanup), and improves circadian rhythm alignment. Do not skip breakfast to achieve the early eating window; instead, begin eating breakfast at the same time and finish dinner 12 hours later.

Introduce fermented foods daily. These contain live beneficial bacteria that improve intestinal barrier function and SCFA production. Examples: unsweetened yoghurt or kefir (if dairy-tolerated), sauerkraut, kimchi, miso, tempeh. If fermented foods are new to you, begin with small quantities (1–2 tablespoons) to allow your gut microbiota to adapt. These foods directly support mood and metabolic health through the mechanisms discussed throughout this book.

Removing inflammatory oils and advanced supplementation

Remove seed oils, soybean oil, sunflower oil, safflower oil, canola oil, which are high in omega-6 polyunsaturated fats and have been oxidised during processing and cooking. Replace them with extra-virgin olive oil (for low-heat cooking and dressings), butter or ghee (for cooking at moderate temperatures), and coconut oil (for higher-heat cooking). This switch reduces systemic and neuroinflammation.

Add B-complex vitamins (methylated forms): Methylated B vitamins are more bioavailable and more supportive of methylation-dependent processes. Include B6 (pyridoxal-5-phosphate form), B12 (methylcobalamin or cyanocobalamin), and folate (methylfolate). This supports neurotransmitter synthesis and mental health. Add zinc picolinate (15–25 mg daily with dinner). Zinc supports immune function, metabolic rate, and mood.

Continuous glucose monitoring for personalisation

If accessible, wear a continuous glucose monitor for two weeks. Devices like Freestyle Libre (available through the NHS for those with diabetes, or available privately) provide real-time glucose data and reveal your personal glucose responses to different foods. This feedback is extraordinarily educational: you will see exactly which meals stabilise your glucose and which spike it. This knowledge allows you to personalise your diet based on your individual physiology.

By the end of Week 6, your metabolic function should be noticeably improved. Your energy should be stable, your mood should be substantially more stable, and your mental clarity should be enhanced. You are also beginning to develop the intuitive understanding of how different foods affect your physiology, knowledge that will serve you for life.

Weeks 7–8: Refine and Personalise

Analysing your data and establishing sustainable exercise

If you used a CGM, review your glucose patterns. Identify your three highest-glucose meals and substitute lower-glycaemic alternatives. Use online databases (like the Glycemic Index database, maintained by the University of Sydney) to identify lower-GI alternatives to your favourite foods.

By now, your energy and mood should have improved enough to support more intentional exercise. Establish a routine of 3–4 sessions per week, mixing aerobic exercise (walking, cycling, swimming, running) and resistance training (bodyweight exercises, gym weights, or resistance bands). Exercise directly improves insulin sensitivity, supports mood through endorphin and serotonin release, and improves cardiovascular health. The specific type of exercise matters less than consistency and that you choose activities you enjoy and can sustain.

Addressing remaining deficiencies and assessing progress

Review your baseline test results and the symptoms you have tracked throughout these 8 weeks. If you identified iron deficiency, ferritin supplementation or dietary iron becomes a priority. If B12 levels were borderline, consider intramuscular B12 injections or high-dose sublingual B12. If vitamin D levels were very low, continue supplementing and retest in 3 months.

Track the mental health metrics you care about most. For those with depression, assess mood using a simple scale (0–10) several times per week. For those with anxiety, track anxiety levels and note when they are highest and lowest. For those with PTSD, track intrusive thoughts and hyperarousal symptoms. For those with bipolar disorder, track mood stability and sleep. By Week 8, you should see meaningful improvement in these metrics. This improvement is the biological reward that reinforces the behavioural changes you have made.

Your three options at Week 8

Continue and deepen the current protocol: For many readers, the 8-week protocol produces such marked improvement that the motivation to continue is organic. You might deepen the protocol by incorporating a Mediterranean diet (as discussed in previous chapters), investigating intermittent fasting, or continuing CGM to further personalise your dietary choices.

Investigate ketogenic metabolic therapy: If you are struggling with treatment-resistant depression, bipolar disorder, or other serious conditions, the 8-week protocol might be a foundation upon which to build a more targeted ketogenic approach. Work with a clinician experienced in ketogenic metabolic therapy to safely transition into this more specialised intervention.

Seek professional support: If progress has been modest, or if you have identified significant deficiencies or dysregulations through your baseline testing, seek consultation with a registered dietitian, metabolic psychiatry specialist, or functional medicine practitioner. These professionals can provide personalised guidance based on your unique biology, medication interactions, and circumstances.

Managing Common Obstacles: Solutions for Real Life

Energy crashes despite protein breakfast: Increase fat at breakfast (add butter, olive oil, or avocado); ensure the carbohydrate component is truly complex (steel-cut oats, not instant oats). Verify sleep is consistent and at least 7 hours. Consider chromium picolinate 200 μg twice daily.

Intense sugar cravings despite stable diet: Increase magnesium supplementation to 400–500 mg daily; add chromium picolinate 200 μg twice daily. Identify the trigger for cravings (stress? boredom? afternoon fatigue?). Have a protein snack ready (handful of nuts, hard-boiled egg, protein shake).

Sleep still disrupted: Ensure last meal is at least 3 hours before bed and is balanced (protein + fat, not carbohydrate-heavy). Eliminate alcohol (at least temporarily), it disrupts sleep architecture. Assess for sleep apnoea symptoms and screen with your GP. Add magnesium threonate (which crosses the blood-brain barrier) in addition to magnesium glycinate.

No mood improvement by Week 4: Obtain full baseline bloodwork if not already done. Ensure B12, folate, iron, and vitamin D are being actively supplemented. Screen thyroid function. Consider SIBO testing if abdominal bloating or irregular stools persist. Review medications for nutrient depletions (e.g., metformin depletes B12, statins deplete CoQ10).

Exercise feels exhausting: Test ferritin and B12; if deficient, supplement aggressively. Ensure you are eating adequate protein (1.2–1.6 grams per kilogram of bodyweight daily). Reduce exercise frequency to 2–3 sessions per week if currently doing more; allow recovery. Ensure sleep is adequate.

Weight loss stalls: Increase resistance exercise; consider a modest calorie deficit (10–15 per cent below maintenance) while ensuring adequate protein. Verify stress management and sleep. Test thyroid function; if TSH is elevated, verify medication dosing.

Tracking Your Progress: Simple Daily Markers

You cannot manage what you do not measure. The following simple daily tracking creates metabolic literacy, the understanding of how different foods, sleep, stress, and movement patterns affect your physiology and mood. You do not need fancy apps; a notebook or simple phone notes suffice.

Each morning, upon waking, rate your energy on a scale of 1–10 and your sleep quality the previous night (1–10). Note any dreams recalled. These simple metrics reveal whether your nervous system is regulating correctly, poor sleep and low morning energy suggest ongoing dysglycaemia or HPA axis dysregulation.

Post-meal (1–2 hours after lunch and dinner), note your mood (1–10) and energy (1–10). Also note your hunger at the next scheduled meal. If you are ravenous 2–3 hours after eating despite a balanced meal, this suggests your meal was too high in carbohydrate or too low in fat or protein. If you are not hungry at the next meal, this suggests satiety is good.

Each evening, rate your mood stability across the day (1–10), rate any anxiety or mood swings experienced, and note your sleep quality and restfulness. Note any significant stressors or emotional events.

Weekly, note any changes in overall anxiety level, concentration, emotional reactivity, and mood. Also track any physical changes: skin clarity, energy, digestion (bloating? regularity?), or weight/how clothes fit. Over time, this simple tracking reveals patterns invisible in the moment: you might notice that days after poor sleep, your glucose spikes are larger and your mood is more reactive. You might notice that meals with a particular food are followed by afternoon anxiety, while other meals leave you stable. You might notice that days with exercise are followed by deeper sleep. These personal metabolic insights are more powerful than any generic recommendation, they create intrinsic motivation to maintain the practices that work for your unique biology.

Working with Your Healthcare Team

This book provides a framework, not a prescription. If you are taking psychiatric medications, blood sugar-regulating medications, or other chronic medications, share the relevant chapters with your GP, psychiatrist, or community mental health team. The metabolic psychiatry approach works best as a complement to, not replacement for, professional mental health care. Your clinician may have important insights about which interventions are safe for you specifically, particularly regarding medication-nutrient interactions.

Additionally, the landscape of metabolic psychiatry is changing rapidly. An increasing number of clinicians, psychiatrists, GPs, and nurse practitioners, are being trained in metabolic approaches to mental illness. If your current clinician is unfamiliar with this framework, you might seek a second opinion from a practitioner trained in this area. Organisations like the International Society of Nutritional Psychiatry Research and the Metabolic Psychiatry Institute maintain registries of trained clinicians. The goal is integration: conventional psychiatric care that addresses neurotransmitter dysfunction, psychological trauma, and social stressors, working in partnership with metabolic interventions that address the blood sugar stability and microbiome health that underlie and perpetuate psychiatric illness. This integrated approach, meeting the person where they are, using all available evidence-based tools, offers the most complete and durable path to mental health recovery.

Key Takeaways

- Baseline testing (fasting glucose, fasting insulin, HbA1c, vitamin D, B12, folate, magnesium, thyroid) provides the information needed to personalise your metabolic protocol.
- Weeks 1–2 focus on removing the most disruptive foods (liquid sugars, refined carbohydrates) and establishing sleep and meal timing; expect rapid improvements.
- Weeks 3–4 build structural meal composition (the plate method) and introduce vitamin D3 and omega-3 supplementation.
- Weeks 5–6 deepen the protocol with time-restricted eating, microbiome restoration, and advanced supplementation (methylated B vitamins, zinc).

- Weeks 7–8 refine based on your personal response, establish sustainable exercise, and decide on next steps (continue, deepen, or seek professional support).
- Simple daily tracking (energy, mood, sleep, hunger, digestion) creates metabolic literacy and reveals which practices work best for your unique biology.

Next Steps: Your Metabolic Recovery Journey

You have now completed an 8-week metabolic reset. The science underlying each intervention has been explained. The evidence supporting each dietary change, supplement, and lifestyle practice has been presented throughout this book. What remains is your choice: to integrate these practices into your daily life, to develop the resilience and agency that comes from understanding how your metabolism directly shapes your mind, and to claim the mental health that is your biological birthright.

The goal is not perfection. The goal is not to achieve a flawlessly stable glucose line or to eliminate all processed food from your life permanently. The goal is to develop awareness, build sustainable habits, and make incremental improvements that, compounded over months and years, add up to measurably better mental health, greater resilience, and a richer, more energetic life. You have more control over your mental health through lifestyle choices than the current medical model typically acknowledges. This 8-week protocol, and the 32 chapters preceding it, is an invitation to exercise that control. Begin where you are. Use what you have. Do what you can. Your metabolic recovery, and the mental health that follows, is possible.

References

Craft, S., Baker, L. D., Montine, T. J., Donohoe, S., Harless, K., Sharp, D., ... & Plymate, S. R. (2012). Intranasal insulin therapy for age-related cognitive decline: A randomised, double-blind, placebo-controlled trial. *Archives of Neurology*, 69(1), 29–38. https://doi.org/10.1001/archneurol.2011.233

Estruch, R., Ros, E., Salas-Salvadó, J., Covas, M. I., Corella, D., Arós, F., … & Martínez-González, M. A. (2013). Primary prevention of cardiovascular disease with a Mediterranean diet. *New England Journal of Medicine*, 368(14), 1279–1290. https://doi.org/10.1056/NEJMoa1200303

Mozaffarian, D., Benjamin, E. J., Go, A. S., Arnett, D. K., Blaha, M. J., Cushman, M., ... & Turner, M. B. (2016). Heart disease and stroke statistics,2016 update: A report from the American Heart Association. *Circulation*, 133(4), e38–e360. https://doi.org/10.1161/CIR.0000000000000350

Porges, S. W. (2001). The polyvagal theory: Phylogenetic substrates of a social nervous system. *International Journal of Psychophysiology*, 42(2), 123–146. https://doi.org/10.1016/S0167-8760(01)00162-3

Russell, M. E. B., Scott, A. B., Boggero, I. A., & Carlson, C. R. (2017). Inclusion of a rest period in diaphragmatic breathing increases high frequency heart rate variability: Implications for behavioral therapy. *Psychophysiology*, 54(3), 358–365. https://doi.org/10.1111/psyp.12798

Zeevi, D., Korem, T., Zmora, N., Israeli, D., Rothschild, D., Weinberger, A., ... & Elinav, E. (2015). Personalized nutrition by prediction of glycaemic responses. *Cell*, 163(5), 1079–1094. https://doi.org/10.1016/j.cell.2015.11.001

Chapter 34: Medications, Metabolism, and Mental Health

Introduction: If you are reading this book whilst taking psychiatric medication, you belong to a very large group. Globally, antidepressants, antipsychotics, and mood stabilisers are among the most commonly prescribed drugs, and in Australia, antidepressant use has doubled over the past two decades. This chapter is not an argument against medication. For many people, psychiatric medication is life-saving, it reduces the severity of symptoms enough to function, engage in therapy, and begin rebuilding. Rather, this chapter addresses something that is rarely discussed in the medication conversation: the significant metabolic effects of many psychiatric drugs and what you can do to protect your physical health whilst taking them. Understanding the relationship between your medication and your blood sugar is not a reason to stop your medication. It is a reason to be better informed and more proactive about metabolic monitoring.

Why This Matters: The Metabolic Side-Effect Gap

When psychiatrists prescribe antipsychotics, mood stabilisers, or antidepressants, the informed consent conversation typically focuses on psychiatric side effects, sedation, sexual dysfunction, weight gain as a general warning. What is rarely discussed in detail is the specific metabolic mechanism by which many of these medications disrupt glucose regulation and why that matters for both physical and mental health.

The irony is this: several of the medications most commonly used to treat mood disorders create physiological conditions, insulin resistance, chronic low-grade inflammation, dysbiosis, that independently worsen mood, energy, and cognition. Addressing these metabolic effects is not an optional extra. It is central to achieving the best possible outcome from treatment.

Atypical Antipsychotics: The Metabolic Challenge

The atypical (second-generation) antipsychotics represent perhaps the most significant metabolic challenge in psychiatric pharmacology. Medications including olanzapine (Zyprexa), clozapine (Clozaril), quetiapine (Seroquel), and risperidone (Risperdal) have well-documented associations with weight gain, insulin resistance, elevated fasting glucose, dyslipidaemia (raised triglycerides, lowered HDL cholesterol), and new-onset type 2 diabetes.

The mechanisms are multiple. These medications block histamine H1 receptors, powerfully stimulating appetite and promoting weight gain independently of caloric intake. They antagonise serotonin 5-HT2C receptors, further increasing appetite and carbohydrate cravings specifically. Some directly impair pancreatic beta-cell function and insulin sensitivity independent of weight gain, a particularly concerning finding, as it means metabolic effects cannot be entirely attributed to weight change.

The scale of these effects is clinically significant. Studies show that up to 40 per cent of individuals taking olanzapine long-term develop metabolic syndrome, and the risk of new-onset type 2 diabetes is approximately three to four times higher in patients taking atypical antipsychotics compared to the general population. Clozapine and olanzapine carry the highest metabolic risk; aripiprazole (Abilify) and ziprasidone (Zeldox) carry lower risk; quetiapine and risperidone are intermediate.

This does not mean these medications should be avoided, for conditions such as schizophrenia, bipolar disorder with psychotic features, and treatment-resistant depression, they are often the most effective available treatment. It means their metabolic effects must be actively monitored and managed.

Mood Stabilisers: Lithium, Valproate, and Metabolic Health

Lithium remains one of the most effective mood stabilisers available for bipolar disorder, but it has a complex metabolic profile. Long-term lithium use is associated with weight gain (5–10 kg on average), hypothyroidism (in up to 40 per cent of long-term users), and impaired renal concentrating ability. Hypothyroidism itself worsens depression, fatigue, and cognitive function, creating a scenario where the medication treating bipolar disorder is simultaneously driving a condition that mimics depressive episodes. Regular thyroid monitoring is essential for anyone on lithium.

Valproate (sodium valproate, Epilim) is associated with significant weight gain and insulin resistance. Studies suggest valproate increases appetite through effects on GABA pathways whilst potentially impairing mitochondrial fatty acid oxidation. Women taking valproate face additional concerns: the drug is associated with polycystic ovarian syndrome (PCOS), a condition characterised by insulin resistance, elevated androgens, and ovulatory dysfunction. For women of reproductive age on valproate, gynaecological monitoring and attention to insulin sensitivity is especially important.

Lamotrigine (Lamictal), which is effective for bipolar depression and increasingly used as an augmentation agent, has a more metabolically neutral profile and may be preferable where clinically appropriate.

Antidepressants: Mixed Metabolic Signals

The metabolic picture for antidepressants is more nuanced. SSRIs (selective serotonin reuptake inhibitors) have generally been considered metabolically neutral or even mildly beneficial, some studies suggest they modestly reduce insulin resistance and improve glycaemic control. However, weight gain is documented with long-term SSRI use (particularly with paroxetine and escitalopram), and some research suggests that chronic SSRI use may alter glucose metabolism in complex ways.

Tricyclic antidepressants (TCAs), amitriptyline, nortriptyline, clomipramine, carry more significant metabolic risks: pronounced weight gain, increased insulin resistance, and elevated triglycerides. Their antihistaminergic and anticholinergic properties drive appetite stimulation and carbohydrate cravings similar (though less potent) to those seen with antipsychotics. SNRIs (serotonin-noradrenaline reuptake inhibitors) such as venlafaxine and duloxetine have variable effects; venlafaxine in particular has been associated with elevated blood pressure and increased fasting glucose in some studies.

Mirtazapine (Avanza, Remeron), a widely used atypical antidepressant, has significant antihistaminergic properties and is associated with substantial weight gain and metabolic disruption in long-term use. Its appetite-stimulating effects are sometimes used therapeutically in patients who need weight gain, but they present a challenge for individuals already managing insulin resistance.

Practical Strategies: Protecting Metabolic Health on Psychiatric Medication

Understanding the metabolic effects of your medication is the first step. What follows are evidence-based strategies to protect metabolic health without compromising psychiatric treatment.

Monitor regularly. Current guidelines recommend baseline metabolic testing before starting antipsychotics and at least annual reassessment: fasting glucose, HbA1c, fasting lipid panel, weight, waist circumference, and blood pressure. In practice, these guidelines are inconsistently followed. Be your own advocate: ask your GP or psychiatrist to include metabolic monitoring as part of your regular reviews. Request fasting glucose, HbA1c, and a lipid panel at least annually.

Prioritise diet quality. The dietary principles in this book, stable blood sugar, adequate protein, dietary fibre, anti-inflammatory foods, limited refined carbohydrates and sugars, are especially important for individuals on metabolically active psychiatric medications. Dietary improvements cannot completely counteract medication-induced metabolic effects, but they meaningfully reduce their severity. Several studies have shown that structured dietary intervention reduces weight gain and insulin resistance in patients taking antipsychotics.

Exercise matters more, not less. Regular physical activity, particularly resistance training, improves insulin sensitivity and helps offset medication-induced metabolic disruption. A 2014 systematic review found that structured exercise programmes significantly reduced metabolic syndrome severity in patients on antipsychotics. Resistance training is particularly effective at improving insulin sensitivity and maintaining muscle mass; even two sessions per week have measurable benefits.

Consider metformin where appropriate. Metformin, typically used in type 2 diabetes management, has an evidence base for reducing antipsychotic-induced weight gain and improving insulin sensitivity in psychiatric patients. A Cochrane review found that metformin reduced antipsychotic-induced weight gain by an average of 3 kg compared to placebo. This is a conversation to have with your prescriber if you are experiencing significant metabolic effects on antipsychotic therapy.

Support gut health actively. Atypical antipsychotics have been shown to alter the gut microbiome in ways that promote weight gain and insulin resistance, partly through effects on Lactobacillus and Akkermansia species. Active gut health support, fermented foods, prebiotic fibre, a quality probiotic, may partially mitigate these microbiome-mediated metabolic effects.

Review medication options with your prescriber. If metabolic effects are severe and compromising physical health, a conversation with your prescribing doctor about whether an alternative medication with a lower metabolic burden might achieve similar psychiatric outcomes is entirely appropriate. Never stop or reduce psychiatric medication without medical guidance, abrupt discontinuation can cause serious withdrawal effects and psychiatric relapse.

How to Talk to Your Doctor

Many people feel reluctant to raise concerns about their medication's side effects, fearing they will be perceived as non-compliant or ungrateful. This is understandable but misplaced. Your physical health is as much a clinical priority as your psychiatric health, and a good prescriber will welcome an informed conversation.

You might say: "I've been reading about the metabolic effects of [medication name] and I'd like to understand my personal risk and what we should be monitoring. Can we include metabolic blood tests in my next review?" Or: "I've been putting on weight and I'm concerned about my blood sugar. Are there dietary or lifestyle approaches that might help, and should we consider any alternatives with a lower metabolic burden?"

Bring your own data: your mood and energy tracking, your food diary, any bloodwork you have had recently. The more information you can provide, the better the conversation can be.

A Note on the Broader Picture

The goal of this chapter is not to create anxiety about psychiatric medication, but to illuminate a dimension of metabolic health that is often overlooked. Psychiatric medications help millions of people lead fuller lives. The task is to manage their metabolic effects proactively, so that the physical costs of treatment are minimised. In the ideal scenario, as metabolic health improves through the interventions in this book, some individuals may find, in collaboration with their prescribing doctor, that lower doses of medication are sufficient, or that certain medications can eventually be tapered. This is a conversation to have over time, with clinical guidance, not a goal to pursue unilaterally.

Key Takeaways

- Many psychiatric medications, particularly atypical antipsychotics and some mood stabilisers, cause significant metabolic side effects including weight gain, insulin resistance, dyslipidaemia, and new-onset type 2 diabetes.
- Olanzapine and clozapine carry the highest metabolic risk among antipsychotics; aripiprazole and ziprasidone carry lower risk.
- Valproate is associated with weight gain, insulin resistance, and risk of polycystic ovarian syndrome in women.
- Lithium requires regular thyroid monitoring, as hypothyroidism is a common long-term consequence.
- Antidepressants have variable metabolic effects; TCAs and mirtazapine carry more risk than most SSRIs.
- Practical protective strategies include regular metabolic monitoring, dietary improvement, regular resistance exercise, gut health support, and discussing metformin with your prescriber where weight gain is significant.
- Never stop or reduce psychiatric medication without medical guidance; the metabolic conversation belongs within your ongoing clinical care.

Next Steps

If you are taking psychiatric medication, book a review appointment with your GP in the next month and specifically request a metabolic screen: fasting glucose, HbA1c, fasting lipids, and thyroid function if on lithium. Bring the information from this chapter to that appointment. Begin the dietary and lifestyle strategies outlined in Chapter 33, they are relevant and important regardless of your medication status, and the evidence suggests they meaningfully reduce medication-induced metabolic disruption. Your physical and mental health are not separate concerns, they are the same concern.

References

De Hert, M., Detraux, J., van Winkel, R., Yu, W., & Correll, C. U. (2011). Metabolic and cardiovascular adverse effects associated with antipsychotic drugs. *Nature Reviews Endocrinology*, 8(2), 114–126. https://doi.org/10.1038/nrendo.2011.156

Newcomer, J. W. (2007). Antipsychotic medications: Metabolic and cardiovascular risk. *Journal of Clinical Psychiatry*, *68*(Suppl 4), 8–13. PMID: 17539694

Correll, C. U., Detraux, J., De Lepeleire, J., & De Hert, M. (2015). Effects of antipsychotics, antidepressants and mood stabilizers on risk for physical diseases in people with schizophrenia, depression and bipolar disorder. *World Psychiatry*, 14(2), 119–136. https://doi.org/10.1002/wps.20204

Álvarez-Jiménez, M., Hetrick, S. E., González-Blanch, C., Gleeson, J. F., & McGorry, P. D. (2008). Non-pharmacological management of antipsychotic-induced weight gain: Systematic review and meta-analysis of randomised controlled trials. *British Journal of Psychiatry*, 193(2), 101–107. https://doi.org/10.1192/bjp.bp.107.042853

Wu, R. R., Zhao, J. P., Jin, H., Shao, P., Fang, M. S., Guo, X. F., He, Y. Q., Liu, Y. J., Chen, J. D., & Li, L. H. (2008). Lifestyle intervention and metformin for treatment of antipsychotic-induced weight gain. *JAMA*, 299(2), 185–193. https://doi.org/10.1001/jama.2007.56-a

Firth, J., Stubbs, B., Rosenbaum, S., Vancampfort, D., Malchow, B., Schuch, F., Elliott, R., Nuechterlein, K. H., & Yung, A. R. (2017). Aerobic exercise improves cognitive functioning in people with schizophrenia: A systematic review and meta-analysis. *Schizophrenia Bulletin*, 43(3), 546–556. https://doi.org/10.1093/schbul/sbw115

Morgan, A. J., & Jorm, A. F. (2008). Self-help interventions for depressive disorders and depressive symptoms: A systematic review. *Annals of General Psychiatry*, 7, 13. https://doi.org/10.1186/1744-859X-7-13

Maayan, L., Vakhrusheva, J., & Correll, C. U. (2010). Effectiveness of medications used to attenuate antipsychotic-related weight gain and metabolic abnormalities: A systematic review and meta-analysis. *Neuropsychopharmacology*, 35(7), 1520–1530. https://doi.org/10.1038/npp.2010.21

Zheng, W., Zhang, Q. E., Cai, D. B., Yang, X. H., Qiu, Y., Ungvari, G. S., Ng, C. H., Ning, Y. P., Wang, G., & Xiang, Y. T. (2019). Augmentation of metformin for antipsychotic-induced weight gain and metabolic syndrome: A meta-analysis. *Journal of Affective Disorders*, 250, 38–46. https://doi.org/10.1016/j.jad.2019.02.049

Morgan, V. A., McGrath, J. J., Jablensky, A., Badcock, J. C., Waterreus, A., Bush, R., Carr, V., Castle, D., Cohen, M., Galletly, C., Harvey, C., Hocking, B., McGorry, P., Neil, A. L., Saw, S., Shah, S., Stain, H. J., & Mackinnon, A. (2014). Psychosis prevalence and physical, behavioural and socio-economic co-morbidities in an Australian population. *Australian and New Zealand Journal of Psychiatry*, 48(5), 416–424. https://doi.org/10.1177/0004867413512355

Glossary

Adrenal fatigue / HPA axis dysregulation

A state where the adrenal glands struggle to produce adequate cortisol and other stress hormones due to chronic stress, poor nutrition, or sleep disruption. This condition involves dysregulation of the hypothalamic-pituitary-adrenal (HPA) axis, which normally coordinates stress responses. Symptoms include fatigue, difficulty concentrating, and increased anxiety. Restoring sleep, nutrition, and stress management can support recovery.

Allostatic load

The cumulative physiological wear and tear on the body from chronic stress and repeated activation of stress response systems. High allostatic load is associated with increased inflammation, insulin resistance, and accelerated ageing. Blood sugar dysregulation is a key contributor to allostatic load. Lifestyle interventions that stabilise blood sugar can reduce this burden on the body.

Blood-brain barrier

A selective membrane that controls which substances pass from the bloodstream into the brain and cerebrospinal fluid. It protects the brain from pathogens and toxins but also requires specific transporters for nutrients like glucose, amino acids, and omega-3 fatty acids. Chronic inflammation can compromise the integrity of the blood-brain barrier. This breakdown may contribute to neuroinflammation and mental health conditions.

Chronobiology / circadian rhythm

The study of biological rhythms and the internal 24-hour cycles that regulate sleep-wake patterns, hormone release, body temperature, and digestion. The circadian rhythm is entrained by light exposure, meal timing, and physical activity. Disruption of circadian rhythms through irregular sleep or eating patterns impairs metabolic health and mood regulation. Aligning daily habits with natural circadian patterns supports mental health and blood sugar stability.

Cortisol

A steroid hormone produced by the adrenal glands in response to stress and regulated by the HPA axis. Cortisol mobilises glucose and suppresses the immune system to prepare for fight-or-flight responses. Elevated or dysregulated cortisol levels promote blood sugar dysregulation, inflammation, and anxiety. Chronic stress leads to cortisol dysregulation, which perpetuates mental health challenges.

Dawn phenomenon

An early-morning rise in blood glucose that occurs before waking, triggered by a surge in cortisol and growth hormone. This can be marked in people with insulin resistance or type 2 diabetes. The dawn phenomenon is exacerbated by poor sleep quality and evening blood sugar dysregulation. Managing evening carbohydrate intake and sleep quality can help minimise this effect.

Dysbiosis

An imbalance in the composition of the gut microbiota, characterised by reduced microbial diversity and overgrowth of pathogenic species. Dysbiosis is often caused by poor diet, antibiotic use, chronic stress, or insufficient sleep. This microbial imbalance increases intestinal permeability and neuroinflammation, both linked to mood disorders. Dietary fibre, fermented foods, and stress management help restore healthy microbial balance.

Endocannabinoid system

An internal signalling system that regulates mood, appetite, pain perception, immune function, and stress responses through cannabinoid receptors throughout the nervous system and gut. Endocannabinoids like anandamide are produced by the body and modulated by omega-3 fatty acids, exercise, and certain foods. Dysregulation of the endocannabinoid system is implicated in depression and anxiety. Supporting this system through lifestyle interventions may improve mental health.

Enteric nervous system

A complex network of approximately 500 million neurons lining the gastrointestinal tract, often called the "second brain." The enteric nervous system controls digestion, nutrient absorption, and gut motility independently but communicates extensively with the central nervous system via the vagus nerve. Dysregulation of the enteric nervous system contributes to both gastrointestinal and mental health problems. Supporting gut health through diet and stress management benefits both systems.

Epigenetics

The study of how environmental factors, including diet, stress, sleep, and toxin exposure, alter gene expression without changing the underlying DNA sequence. Epigenetic changes can be reversed through lifestyle modifications, suggesting that genes are not fixed determinants of health. Poor nutrition and chronic stress promote epigenetic changes associated with mental health disorders. Therapeutic diet and lifestyle changes can restore healthier epigenetic patterns.

Free radicals / oxidative stress

Unstable molecules with unpaired electrons that damage cellular structures, proteins, and DNA by stealing electrons from healthy cells. Oxidative stress occurs when the body's antioxidant defences are overwhelmed by excessive free radical production from inflammation, poor diet, or environmental toxins. Blood sugar dysregulation increases oxidative stress in the brain, contributing to cognitive decline and mood disorders. Antioxidant-rich foods reduce oxidative stress and support neurological health.

GABA (gamma-aminobutyric acid)

The primary inhibitory neurotransmitter in the brain that promotes relaxation, reduces neuronal excitability, and supports sleep and anxiety regulation. GABA is synthesised from glutamate with the help of vitamin B6 and is produced by intestinal bacteria. Dysregulation of GABA signalling is implicated in anxiety and sleep disorders. Supporting GABA production through adequate B vitamins, gut health, and stress management is important for mental wellbeing.

Gluconeogenesis

The metabolic pathway in which the liver produces new glucose from precursors such as amino acids, lactate, and glycerol, primarily during fasting or low-carbohydrate periods. This process is activated by cortisol and glucagon when blood glucose is depleted. While gluconeogenesis provides necessary glucose during fasting, chronic overactivation can impair blood sugar regulation and contribute to reactive hypoglycaemia. Supporting stable blood sugar reduces reliance on excessive gluconeogenesis.

Glycaemic index / glycaemic load

Measures of how quickly and to what extent a food raises blood glucose levels: the glycaemic index rates individual foods on a scale (0–100), whilst glycaemic load accounts for portion size. Foods with a high glycaemic index or load cause rapid blood sugar spikes followed by crashes. These blood sugar fluctuations impair mood, energy, and cognitive function. Choosing lower glycaemic index foods supports sustained energy and mental health.

HbA1c (glycated haemoglobin)

A form of haemoglobin that binds to glucose; HbA1c levels reflect average blood glucose concentrations over the preceding 2–3 months. HbA1c is a key diagnostic marker for prediabetes and diabetes and is now widely recognised as relevant to mental health assessment. Elevated HbA1c correlates with increased risk of depression, anxiety, and cognitive decline. Monitoring HbA1c and implementing dietary changes can improve both metabolic and mental health.

Hippocampal neurogenesis

The birth of new neurons in the hippocampus, a brain region critical for memory formation and emotional regulation. Neurogenesis is supported by exercise, omega-3 fatty acids, meditation, and stable blood glucose levels. Depression is associated with reduced hippocampal neurogenesis; conversely, lifestyle interventions that stabilise blood sugar and reduce inflammation promote neurogenesis. Supporting hippocampal neurogenesis is a mechanism by which metabolic health improves mental health.

Hyperglycaemia / hypoglycaemia

Hyperglycaemia refers to elevated blood glucose levels; hypoglycaemia refers to abnormally low blood glucose levels. Both states trigger stress hormone release and impair cognitive and emotional function. Recurrent hypoglycaemic episodes produce anxiety, irritability, and brain fog; chronic hyperglycaemia promotes inflammation and neurodegeneration. Maintaining stable blood glucose through appropriate nutrition and meal timing prevents both states.

Hypothalamic-pituitary-adrenal (HPA) axis

The primary biological system that regulates stress responses and coordinates the production of cortisol and other stress hormones. The HPA axis links the brain (hypothalamus and pituitary) to the adrenal glands via hormonal signals. Chronic stress and poor metabolic health lead to HPA axis dysregulation, characterised by abnormal cortisol rhythms and impaired stress resilience. Dietary and lifestyle interventions that stabilise blood sugar support healthy HPA axis function.

Inflammasome

A multiprotein complex within immune cells that activates inflammatory responses when triggered by pathogens, cellular damage, or metabolic dysfunction. Dysbiosis, lipopolysaccharides (LPS), and high blood glucose activate inflammasomes, triggering the release of inflammatory cytokines. Inflammasome activation in the brain drives neuroinflammation and mood disorders. Anti-inflammatory dietary and lifestyle approaches reduce inflammasome activation.

Insulin resistance / insulin sensitivity

Insulin resistance occurs when cells fail to respond adequately to insulin, requiring higher insulin levels to maintain normal blood glucose; insulin sensitivity is the inverse, cells respond effectively to lower insulin levels. Insulin resistance develops from chronic consumption of refined carbohydrates, excess weight, and sedentary lifestyle. Insulin resistance impairs glucose delivery to the brain and increases inflammation, contributing to depression and cognitive decline. Dietary changes that restore insulin sensitivity improve mental health.

Intestinal permeability ("leaky gut")

A state in which the intestinal barrier becomes excessively permeable, allowing partially digested food, bacterial endotoxins (LPS), and other antigens to cross into the bloodstream. Common causes include dysbiosis, inflammatory foods, chronic stress, and non-steroidal anti-inflammatory drugs (NSAIDs). Increased intestinal permeability triggers systemic and neuroinflammation, linking gut dysfunction to anxiety, depression, and brain fog. Restoring the intestinal barrier through targeted nutrition and stress management supports mental health recovery.

Ketosis / ketogenic

Ketosis is a metabolic state in which the body burns fat for fuel and produces ketone bodies as an alternative to glucose; a ketogenic diet is high in fat, moderate in protein, and very low in carbohydrates. Ketones provide sustained energy for the brain and have neuroprotective properties that may benefit mood and cognition. Ketogenic approaches can improve blood sugar stability and reduce inflammation in some individuals. However, they require careful implementation and monitoring by healthcare practitioners.

Lipopolysaccharides (LPS)

Endotoxins found in the outer membrane of gram-negative bacteria in the gut that can trigger immune activation and inflammation when they cross the intestinal barrier. Dysbiosis and intestinal permeability increase circulating LPS ("metabolic endotoxaemia"), activating inflammasomes and promoting neuroinflammation. High LPS levels are associated with depression and anxiety. Restoring microbial balance and intestinal barrier function reduces LPS-driven inflammation.

Metabolic syndrome

A cluster of metabolic abnormalities including insulin resistance, elevated blood pressure, abdominal obesity, elevated triglycerides, and reduced HDL cholesterol. Metabolic syndrome significantly increases risk of type 2 diabetes and cardiovascular disease and is strongly associated with depression and anxiety. The condition reflects fundamental dysregulation of glucose and fat metabolism. Comprehensive dietary and lifestyle interventions that restore insulin sensitivity address the root cause of metabolic syndrome.

Microbiome / microbiota

The microbiota refers to the trillions of microorganisms (bacteria, viruses, fungi, archaea) inhabiting the human body, predominantly in the gut; the microbiome is the collective genome of these organisms. The gut microbiota performs essential functions including nutrient synthesis, immune education, and production of neurotransmitters and short-chain fatty acids. Dysbiosis impairs these functions and contributes to both metabolic and mental health problems. Supporting microbial diversity through fibre-rich whole foods underpins health.

Mitochondria / mitochondrial dysfunction

Mitochondria are cellular organelles that generate ATP, the energy currency of cells; mitochondrial dysfunction occurs when energy production is impaired. Blood sugar dysregulation, oxidative stress, and inflammation impair mitochondrial function, reducing cellular energy availability. Mitochondrial dysfunction in brain cells contributes to depression, anxiety, brain fog, and neurodegenerative conditions. Restoring metabolic health through proper nutrition and exercise restores mitochondrial function.

Myelin / myelination

Myelin is a fatty insulating sheath that wraps around axons and enables rapid electrical transmission of nerve impulses; myelination is the process of forming this sheath. Adequate omega-3 fatty acids, cholesterol, and B vitamins are essential for myelin formation and maintenance. Neuroinflammation and blood sugar dysregulation impair myelination, slowing neural transmission and contributing to cognitive dysfunction. Supporting myelin health is important for brain function and mental health.

Neuroinflammation

Chronic low-grade inflammation within the brain and nervous system, triggered by activation of microglial cells and excessive release of pro-inflammatory cytokines. Neuroinflammation is driven by systemic inflammation, dysbiosis, intestinal permeability, and blood sugar dysregulation. Elevated neuroinflammation is observed in depression, anxiety, bipolar disorder, and cognitive decline. Reducing systemic inflammation through dietary and lifestyle changes reduces neuroinflammation and supports mental health recovery.

Neuroplasticity

The brain's capacity to rewire itself by forming new neural connections and reorganising neural pathways in response to experience, learning, and environmental demands. Neuroplasticity underlies recovery from mental health conditions and the effectiveness of therapeutic interventions. Cognitive therapy, meditation, physical exercise, and metabolic support all leverage neuroplasticity. Understanding neuroplasticity provides hope that brain function and mental health can be restored.

Neurotransmitter

A chemical messenger released by neurons to transmit signals across synapses to other neurons or target cells, regulating mood, cognition, sleep, and appetite. Key neurotransmitters relevant to mental health include serotonin, dopamine, GABA, glutamate, and noradrenaline. Blood sugar dysregulation, nutritional deficiencies, and neuroinflammation impair neurotransmitter synthesis and function. Supporting neurotransmitter production through adequate nutrition and metabolic stability underpins mental health.

Omega-3 fatty acids (EPA, DHA)

Essential polyunsaturated fatty acids: eicosapentaenoic acid (EPA) and docosahexaenoic acid (DHA) are derived primarily from marine sources. Omega-3 fatty acids are structural components of neuronal membranes, support myelin formation, reduce neuroinflammation, and modulate the endocannabinoid system. Deficiency in omega-3 fatty acids is associated with depression, anxiety, and cognitive decline. Adequate omega-3 intake from fish, algae, or high-quality supplements supports brain health and mental wellbeing.

Polyphenols

Plant-derived compounds with antioxidant and anti-inflammatory properties found abundantly in coloured vegetables, berries, herbs, tea, coffee, and red wine. Polyphenols support the growth of beneficial gut bacteria and reduce intestinal permeability. Their antioxidant effects protect neurons from oxidative damage and neuroinflammation. Including a diverse range of colourful plant foods provides polyphenols that support both metabolic and mental health.

Postbiotics / prebiotics / probiotics

Probiotics are beneficial live microorganisms (bacteria or yeasts) that colonise the gut and support health. Prebiotics are indigestible food components (typically fibre) that selectively nourish beneficial bacteria. Postbiotics are beneficial metabolites produced by bacteria, including short-chain fatty acids and other compounds with health effects. Together, these support microbial balance and barrier function; adequate intake from whole foods or supplements improves metabolic and mental health.

Reactive hypoglycaemia

An excessive drop in blood glucose occurring 2–3 hours after consuming high-glycaemic-index carbohydrates or sugary foods, followed by a surge in cortisol and adrenaline. This produces acute symptoms including anxiety, tremor, irritability, and brain fog. Reactive hypoglycaemia perpetuates mood instability and food cravings. Selecting lower-glycaemic foods and including protein and healthy fats with carbohydrates prevents reactive hypoglycaemia.

Short-chain fatty acids (SCFAs)

Metabolites produced when gut bacteria ferment dietary fibre, primarily butyrate, propionate, and acetate. SCFAs nourish intestinal cells, strengthen the intestinal barrier, and cross the blood-brain barrier to reduce neuroinflammation. SCFAs support the production of GABA and other neurotransmitters. Adequate fibre intake supports SCFA production, which is essential for both gut and brain health.

Time-restricted eating / intermittent fasting

Eating patterns that limit food consumption to specific time windows, for example, eating only between 12 and 8 pm, or following a 5:2 pattern (eating normally five days, restricting intake two days). These approaches may improve insulin sensitivity, reduce inflammation, and support metabolic health in some individuals. However, they can worsen blood sugar dysregulation in others, particularly those with a history of disordered eating. Implementation requires individualised assessment and monitoring by a healthcare practitioner.

Vagus nerve

The longest cranial nerve, extending from the brainstem through the neck, chest, and abdomen, connecting the brain to the heart, lungs, and gastrointestinal tract. The vagus nerve is the primary channel of the parasympathetic nervous system, promoting relaxation and digestion. The vagus nerve also transmits signals from the gut microbiota to the brain, influencing mood and behaviour. Vagal tone can be improved through breathing exercises, meditation, and social connection, supporting mental health.

Recommended Resources

Books

- Jacka, F. N. (2019). *Brain Changer: How Diet Can Save Your Mental Health*. Macmillan Australia. The landmark book by the researcher behind the SMILES trial, written for a general audience.

- Perlmutter, D. (2013). *Grain Brain: The Surprising Truth about Wheat, Carbs, and Sugar, Your Brain's Silent Killers*. Little, Brown and Company.

- Amen, D. G. (2008). *Change Your Brain, Change Your Life*. Harmony Books. Evidence-based guide to brain health through lifestyle, nutrition, and targeted supplements.

- Hyman, M. (2020). *Food Fix: How to Save Our Health, Our Economy, Our Communities, and Our Planet*. Little, Brown Spark.

- Blaser, M. J. (2014). *Missing Microbes: How the Overuse of Antibiotics Is Fuelling Our Modern Plagues*. Henry Holt. Essential reading on antibiotic overuse and microbiome disruption.

- Panda, S. (2019). *The Circadian Code: Lose Weight, Supercharge Your Energy, and Transform Your Health from Morning to Midnight*. Rodale Books.

- van der Kolk, B. (2014). *The Body Keeps the Score: Brain, Mind, and Body in the Healing of Trauma*. Viking.

- Doney, G. (2021). *Healing Trauma at the Cellular Level*. The companion volume to this book, exploring the intersection of trauma, nervous system dysregulation, and cellular healing.

Websites and Organisations

- **Beyond Blue Australia**, beyondblue.org.au, Australia's leading mental health support organisation providing information, online programmes, and crisis support.

- **Black Dog Institute**, blackdoginstitute.org.au, Australian research and clinical institute focused on mood disorders, with publicly accessible resources.

- **Mindd Foundation**, mindd.org, Australian charity advancing understanding of the nutrition-behaviour-mental health connection.

- **International Society for Nutritional Psychiatry Research (ISNPR)**, isnpr.org, Global organisation facilitating research and education on nutrition and mental health.

- **Nutritional Psychiatry Network Australia**, nutritionalpsychiatry.net.au, Australian clinician network with a practitioner directory.

- **SMILES Trial Resources**, Search "SMILES trial Jacka" for free access to the landmark randomised trial demonstrating dietary improvement for depression.

Apps and Tools

- **Cronometer** (cronometer.com), Comprehensive nutrition tracking that displays micronutrient intake alongside macros; excellent for identifying nutritional gaps.

- **Bearable** (bearable.app), Symptom and mood tracking app designed for chronic health conditions; allows correlation of diet, sleep, and mood data.

- **Levels** (levelshealth.com), Continuous glucose monitoring integration app providing metabolic scoring and meal insights.

- **Insight Timer** (insighttimer.com), Free meditation app with thousands of guided practices for stress reduction, sleep, and anxiety.

- **Abbott FreeStyle LibreLink**, Companion app for the FreeStyle Libre CGM sensor; available via Australian pharmacies without prescription.

Key Blood Tests to Request from Your GP

- **Fasting blood glucose**, Baseline glucose control; levels above 5.6 mmol/L suggest insulin resistance.

- **HbA1c (glycated haemoglobin)**, Average blood glucose over 2–3 months; important for assessing diabetes risk and mental health correlation.

- **Fasting insulin**, Optimal <5 mIU/L; borderline 5–10 mIU/L; elevated (>10 mIU/L) indicates insulin resistance before glucose rises.

- **Full lipid panel**, Triglycerides and HDL cholesterol are key metabolic markers; elevated triglycerides and low HDL indicate blood sugar dysregulation.

- **High-sensitivity C-reactive protein (hs-CRP)**, Marker of systemic inflammation strongly associated with depression and anxiety.

- **Vitamin B12 and folate**, Essential for neurotransmitter synthesis and mood; deficiency causes depression and cognitive dysfunction.

- **Vitamin D (25-OH)**, Deficiency is epidemic in Australia despite sun exposure and is strongly associated with depression and seasonal mood disorders.

- **Full blood count (FBC)**, Identifies anaemia and infection contributing to fatigue and brain fog.

- **Thyroid function (TSH, free T3, free T4, thyroid antibodies)**, Thyroid dysfunction directly impairs mood, metabolism, and cognition.

- **Magnesium (red blood cell magnesium preferred over serum)**, Essential for over 300 enzymatic reactions including HPA axis regulation and sleep architecture.

A Final Note

The emerging science of blood sugar, metabolic health, and mental well-being represents one of the most striking shifts in how we understand the mind-body connection. The brain is not separate from the body's metabolic systems, it is highly sensitive to them. What we eat, how we sleep, how we move, how we manage stress, and how we support our gut microbiome and hormonal balance all directly shape the neurochemical environment in which our thoughts, moods, and mental health exist.

The 33 chapters in this book have mapped the major pathways through which blood sugar stability supports mental wellness, from the foundational biochemistry of insulin and cortisol, through the practical dietary and lifestyle strategies, to the emerging frontiers of microbiome science, real-time glucose monitoring, hormonal cycle awareness, ketogenic metabolic therapy for treatment-resistant illness, and the metabolic prevention of Alzheimer's disease.

This is not about perfection. The goal is not to achieve a flawlessly stable glucose line or to eliminate all processed food from your life permanently. The goal is to develop awareness, build sustainable habits, and make incremental improvements that, compounded over months and years, add up to measurably better mental health, greater resilience, and a richer, more energetic life.

You have more control over your mental health through lifestyle choices than the current medical model typically acknowledges. This book is an invitation to exercise that control, thoughtfully, compassionately, and with the best available science as your guide.

Greg Doney, 2026

Made in the USA
Monee, IL
08 November 2026

67377463R00173